Headache Relief

By Seymour Diamond, M.D.
With Bill Still and Cynthia Still

MJF BOOKS
NEW YORK

Published by MJF Books
Fine Communications
Two Lincoln Square
60 West 66th Street
New York, NY 10023

Headache Relief
ISBN 1-56731-388-4

Copyright © 1995 by Seymour Diamond, M.D., and William T. Still
Illustrations copyright © 1995 by Dan Burner III

This book has also been published as *The Hormone Headache*.

This edition published by arrangement with IDG Books Worldwide, Inc.

Manufactured in the United States of America on acid-free paper

MJF Books and the MJF colophon are trademarks of Fine Creative Media, Inc.

10   9   8   7   6   5   4   3   2   1

This book is dedicated to the 34 million American women suffering with headaches.

$\mathcal{A}$CKNOWLEDGMENTS

I would like to thank Mary Franklin for her editorial assistance in the preparation of this manuscript. To Nancy Cooperman I would like to express my appreciation for her editorial insight and suggestions and to Ivy Stone for her efforts in securing publication of this book. Also, I would like to thank Elaine Diamond for her forbearance and help during the writing of this text. Finally, I would like to express my gratitude to Dr. and Mrs. Edward Lichten for their assistance in the research of the role of hormones in headaches.

S.D.

We would like to thank our children, William, Dara, and Noah, for their loving patience during the long hours we spent researching and writing this book.

B.S./C.S.

CONTENTS

*I*NTRODUCTION

No matter how you look at it, the statistics are staggering. At any given time, two million Americans are suffering from a headache. And each year, forty-five million of them suffer from headaches long and intense enough to interfere with their work. At least half of these seek medical help for their pain. In desperation, they swallow more than eighteen billion pills per year and pay in excess of four billion dollars in their quest for relief.

Who gets all these headaches? Primarily women. Studies show that more than 75 percent of chronic headache sufferers are female. In other words, in the United States alone about fifteen million women go to the doctor for relief from headache pain each year. Eight million of these women suffer from recurrent migraine headache and are willing to do just about anything to escape their blinding pain.

Although few women realize it, their headaches are directly related to hormones. In one study, 70 percent of women with migraine attacks reported that their headaches began just before or during their periods. Now, for the first time, researchers understand that this particular kind of hormonal headache is caused by fluctuations of the sex hormones that regulate a woman's menstrual cycle.

But it's not just a woman's sex hormones that are responsible for causing head pain. Recent research suggests that dozens of hormones govern the temporary biochemical disorder that causes that head pain. Of these, only a few have been identified and their role in headache studied. Even so, understanding the part these hormones play in the phenomenon we call headache can improve a woman's ability to comprehend and cope with her pain.

Despite such findings, this is the first headache book primarily for women. In *The Hormone Headache*, women can find the answers to questions about the cause and cure of sexual headaches, as well as other headaches caused by pregnancy, the Pill, menopause, puberty, menstruation, and much more.

HEADACHE: THE MYSTERY AILMENT

Modern headache treatment is truly a medical miracle, compared with what the vast majority of people have had to endure throughout history. Severe headache is certainly one of the most mysterious of all human ailments. It is probably safe to say that headaches are humankind's oldest yet least understood medical problem. Archaeological evidence suggests that thousands of years ago Stone Age man cut away tiny segments of the skull to allow the escape of the "evil demons" that were thought to cause head pain.

A Mesopotamian poem dating from between 4000 and 3000 B.C. depicts headaches as a punishment from God:

> *Headache roameth over the desert, blowing like the wind,*
> *Flashing like lightning, it is loosed above and below:*
> *It cutteth off like a reed him who feareth not his god. . . .*
> *This man it hath struck and*
> *Like one with heart disease he staggereth,*
> *Like one bereft of reason he is broken . . .*

During the time of the ancient Egyptian dynasties, it was commonly held that head pains were caused by Tiu, the evil spirit of headache. Migraine headache is described in the oldest complete medical book known to exist, the *Ebers Papyrus*. The ancient text was transcribed around 1550 B.C., but drew from sources as far back as 3700 B.C. It described this type of headache as a "sickness of half the head." A prescription given to King Usaphias of Egypt for his severe headaches is one of the oldest recorded medical remedies: a compress of boiled herbs applied to the head.

Since then every conceivable cure has been tried, from wrapping the head in potatoes or in a hangman's noose to bathing the feet in mustard and farina. In the sixth century, St. Gregory claimed that he'd been relieved of a severe headache by pressing his head to the rail around the sepulcher of the tomb of St. Martin. The early Native Americans consumed the testes of beavers bottled in spirits. Fortunately for beavers, this remedy didn't achieve wide popularity in the rest of the world, but, like many other folk remedies, it may have borne the seed of a sound idea. It has since been found that the foreskin of the beaver secretes a solution that contains a salicylate, perhaps derived from the bark of the trees upon which beavers feed. Aspirin, it should be noted, is a salicylate.

By 460 B.C. Hippocrates, the father of medicine, described unilateral headache in some detail. Of one patient he wrote:

> *Most of the time he seemed to see something shining before him like a light, usually in part of the right eye; at the end of a moment, a violent pain supervened in the right temple, then in all the head and neck . . . vomiting, when it became possible, was able to divert the pain and render it more moderate.*

Five hundred years later, the Greek physician Aretaeus of

Cappadocia (A.D. 30–90) led a revival of Hippocrates' work and added further detail to the condition we now call migraine headache. Because pain from this type of headache was unilateral, that is, it occurred in only one side of the head, he referred to it as *heterocrania*.

> *The pain . . . remains in the half of the head. This is called heterocrania, an illness by no means mild . . . if at any time it sets in acutely, it occasions unseemly and dreadful symptoms . . . nausea, vomiting of bilious matters, collapse of the patient. . . . They flee the light; the darkness soothes their disease; nor can they bear readily to look upon or hear anything disagreeable; their sense of smell is vitiated. Neither does any thing agreeable to smell delight them, and they also have an aversion to fetid things: the patients, moreover, are weary of life, and wish to die. . . .*

Unfortunately, the treatment recommended by Aretaeus of Cappadocia was counter-irritation. He proposed that a patient's head should be shaved, then blistering agents applied to the bare scalp, such as pitch, lemnestis, pellitory, euphorbium, or the juice of the thapsia. The resulting pain on the surface of the head was supposed to make one forget the pain within.

A hundred years later, Galen, the Greek physician who founded experimental physiology, wrote extensively on headache and devised theories to explain its origin. He too was an advocate of counter-irritation, suggesting the application of a live electric fish, known as a torpedo, to the forehead. But he also felt that opium, conium, mandragora, and garlic could be used in the treatment process, as well as bleeding and the application of cold compresses.

Galen is credited with coining the term *hemicrania*. The Romans translated hemicrania into the Latin *hemicranium*. It was later corrupted in low Latin to *hemigranea*, then by successive linguistic shifts to *emigranea*, *migranea*, and *migraina*. The French modified *migrana* to *migraine*, the term now universally accepted.

From the time of Galen and for the next thousand years, advances in headache theory and treatment were few and far between. During the same period, the greatest of Islam's medieval surgeons, Albucasis (Abú-al-Qasim), was prescribing the application of a hot iron to the afflicted area. If the pain did not subside, then surgery was called for. An incision would be made over the temple, and a piece of garlic would be inserted into the hole; tight compresses would be applied for the next fifteen hours. When the dressings were removed the wound would be left alone for two to three days. Salves were then applied until healing occurred.

For the next 700 years, surprisingly few new developments in the treatment of headaches took place. In 1684 the leading British physician of his day, Thomas Willis, proposed for the first time that the cause of migraine headache was due to distention of the blood vessels rather than pain in brain tissue. He correctly noted that a number of factors could trigger a migraine attack, including wine, exposure to the sun, sexual activity, overeating, and oversleeping. He recommended anodynes (pain relievers) and hypnotic drugs (sleep-producing agents) but also endorsed more radical treatments such as enemas, the letting of blood, and the application of leeches, millipedes, or wood lice.

It wasn't until the nineteenth century that cluster headaches were described as distinct from migraine headaches. And finally, in 1868, the first modern treatment for migraine was discovered. Edward Woakers reported the use of ergot, a fungus that grows on rye, to treat hemicrania. Another investigator, a Dr. Eulenburg, reported the use of injections of ergot extract, and later ergostine, to treat five cases of headache in 1887. In 1893, Dr. W. R. Gowers developed the first prophylactic therapy, a mixture of nitroglycerin in one-percent alcohol, known as "Gowers's mixture."

It wasn't until 1925, however, that the Swiss chemist Rothlin isolated ergotamine and introduced it into clinical practice. By the 1930s, thanks to the work of Dr. Harold G. Wolff of Cornell Medical College, ergotamine tartrate became established as the treatment of choice for acute migraine attacks. Dr. Wolff was also the first to propose a vascular theory of migraine, which stated that the initial pre-headache phase consisted of constriction of blood vessels inside the skull, followed by dilation of the blood vessels outside the skull during the attack. Dr. Wolff's work is often cited as the beginning of the modern era in migraine research.

For the next thirty years, ergotamine was the only treatment that had been proven effective against severe, chronic headaches in a significant proportion of patients. Then in 1966 a group of researchers showed that the use of the drug propranolol was also effective in preventing migraine headache. Since then, the number of treatments that have been proven to be effective for severe, chronic headaches has exploded.

In 1986 serotonin receptors were discovered. This finally gave researchers an understanding of how the blood vessels of the brain become inflamed, the first step in a migraine headache attack. The breakthrough soon led to the discovery of the drug sumatriptan (Imitrex), which helps block serotonin, thus preventing the swelling of the blood vessels and the pain of migraine. Now sumatriptan is used extensively in aborting migraine and is being investigated for cluster headache. For preventive therapy doctors are also armed with remedies such as calcium channel blockers, beta blockers, nonsteroidal anti-inflammatory agents, and other serotonin agonists.

Recently nondrug therapies for headache, like biofeedback, are demonstrating how incredibly powerful the mind/body connection really is. Headache sufferers are actually learning to prevent their headaches by gaining conscious control of autonomic body functions such as heart rate and blood pressure.

Despite this new proliferation of treatments, mystery still surrounds the cause of severe, chronic headache. In 1987 researchers Charles Adler, Sheila Morrissey Adler, and Russell Packard wrote:

> *It is astonishing how successful we have been at treating headache without even fully knowing what pain is or being able to accurately define how drugs and other interventions relieve it. The fact that we nonetheless often can efficiently block the pain of headache is, perhaps, as close as we dare come, in the present day, to magic.*

1

WHICH HEADACHE?

I KNOW ALL ABOUT YOU!

Because you are reading this book, I already know a lot about you. I know you are an intelligent woman who is rather self-reliant. You like to weigh all factors carefully before you make a decision, especially about matters concerning your health.

I also know that you suffer from severe, recurrent headaches. I know that because you are taking the time to read a book about them. Finally, I know that many of you are worried. You wonder: What's triggering my headaches? Do I have a brain tumor? Am I about to have a stroke? And most important of all, how do I stop the pain?

You would probably like to ask a doctor these questions, but for any of a variety of reasons you've chosen to read this book instead. Many of you have already been to a doctor, or perhaps several doctors, and gotten little or no relief. That's a shame. The intense pain of a migraine headache is debilitating to the body as well as to the pocketbook. But worst of all, believing that such headaches are incurable crushes the spirit.

It is said that headaches are the most common ailment a family doctor treats. One estimate is that between 50 and 90 percent of all patients complain to their doctor at one time or another about various types of headaches. Although there are different kinds of headaches, some involving constriction and dilation of the blood vessels and some involving muscle tension, hormones are the root cause of many of these changes. Researchers now realize that hormones in one way or another play a central role in all headache pain. Scientists have currently identified about thirty hormones, with new ones being detected all the time. It is likely that many more hormones await discovery, each holding the promise of knowledge that will tell us more about how to prevent or abort headaches.

The good news is that nearly every woman, no matter how long she has suffered from severe, recurrent headaches, can now find significant relief. Once you can figure out what's setting off your headaches, you can almost always bring them under control. Medications, dietary changes, relaxation, and biofeedback techniques can eliminate or reduce more than 90 percent of headaches.

Surprisingly, such success is a very recent development. Until 1966 ergotamine tartrate was the only medication proved to stop a severe headache. But headache treatment has advanced more in the past twenty years than in all of the previous 6,000 years of medical history. Women and their families need to know that it is not necessary to live with headache pain any longer.

Using this chapter carefully should help you identify the type of headache you are suffering. That's important to know because what may improve one type of headache might make another type of headache worse. Doctors generally group the many different kinds of headaches into three basic categories, each with different causes, symptoms, and treatments. These are:

1. Tension-type headaches (common, everyday headache)
2. Vascular headaches
   a. Migraine headaches
   b. Cluster headaches
3. Headaches due to organic causes (such as brain tumors, aneurysms, or inflammation of the blood vessels)

Tension-type headaches caused by muscle contraction are the most common form of headache. At any given time, two million Americans are suffering from this kind of headache. They occur about five times as frequently as migraines, which involve more complicated vascular changes. Besides migraine, headaches of a vascular nature include cluster headaches and toxic vascular headaches.

The term "vascular" refers to the blood vessels. In vascular headaches blood vessel swelling is thought to be the major component in the production of pain. The blood vessels surrounding the brain become distended, causing pain. Vascular headaches are usually throbbing in character, and physical exertion increases the pain.

WOMEN'S CLUSTER HEADACHES

It's been estimated that chronic migraine headaches afflict eight to twelve million Americans. Cluster headaches are far

Anatomy of a Blood Vessel

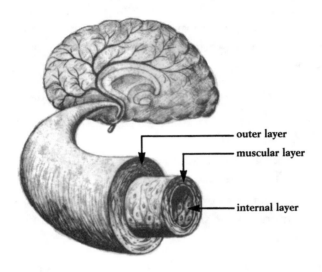

outer layer

muscular layer

internal layer

less prevalent. Interestingly, most migraine sufferers are women, and the vast majority of cluster headache sufferers are men. Cluster headache is a one-sided headache that occurs in a group, series, or bunch of attacks. It typically lasts only a half hour to an hour and causes severe pain, tearing of the eyes, congestion of the nose, and flushing of the face. The Diamond Headache Clinic first reported on a new cluster headache syndrome that occurs primarily in women (*Archives of Neurology* 38:705–709, 1981). Actually, this syndrome is not new but was unrecognized for a number of years. Called the "atypical cluster headache," or "cluster variant headache," it has several unique characteristics. It is chronic and like other cluster headaches can occur several times a day. It is described as atypical because the pain of this kind of cluster headache does not always occur over the eye. They may last all day long, and they can also shift from one location to another.

Women with this type of headache may suffer from many short, jabbing or icepick-like pains in various locations throughout the head. They may also complain of a continuous one-sided headache that throbs and is very intense. Fortunately, women who exhibit at least two or three of these symptoms respond well to a drug used for arthritis, the anti-inflammatory agent indomethacin (Indocin). Fifty percent of sufferers have obtained complete control of the headaches and 80 percent have experienced some relief with the use of indomethacin alone.

TOXIC VASCULAR HEADACHES

Toxic vascular headaches, such as those caused by alcohol-induced hangovers, affect untold millions. Toxic vascular headaches, despite their ominous name, are rarely dangerous. They are caused by something from outside or inside the body, such as infections or chemicals. The most common toxic vascular headache is one caused by a fever accompanying illnesses like the flu, mononucleosis, measles, mumps, pneumonia, or tonsillitis. The pain of such headaches is similar to that of migraine. Medications, like aspirin, that reduce fever will also reduce this type of head pain.

Similarly, the consumption of or exposure to nitrates and nitrites may trigger toxic vascular headaches because they force the blood vessels to swell. Nitrates are found in medications for heart problems and in chemicals used in the munitions industry. Nitrites are also widely used as preservatives in certain processed meats. Monosodium glutamate is another food substance that produces toxic headaches. The same is true of poisons such as lead, benzene, carbon tetrachloride, and insecticides. In addition, trying to quit your caffeine habit "cold turkey," or just missing your morning cup of coffee or tea, can trigger this type of vascular headache.

ORGANIC HEADACHES

Unlike other types of vascular headaches, those due to organic causes are usually very serious. Such headaches are just the tip of the iceberg for dangerous medical conditions, such as brain tumors or strokes, which require immediate medical attention by a skilled specialist. Fortunately, these types of headaches are relatively rare.

MEDICAL HISTORY: THE FIRST STEP TO RELIEF

It's a shame that some doctors commonly prescribe pain-relieving drugs for women's headache conditions without first completing a thorough history, physical exam, and neurological examination. These are standard parts of a thorough examination. Many women undergo exhaustive and risky testing without completing an adequate history of their headache condition. Such an oversight can lead to problems and I certainly don't recommend it.

Even when doctors do perform physical, neurological, and laboratory examinations, the results are often discouragingly normal. For this reason, I'm convinced that the only way to accurately diagnose your headache disorder is by carefully recording the symptoms that characterize your particular problem. Since the key to the diagnosis and treatment of any headache condition is a careful and thorough history, let's just take a minute and jot down a few notes about your symptoms.

Get a pencil and follow along; I've got seventeen questions for you. Check the type of headache that seems to fit your particular symptoms most closely. If it's tough to choose between two or more symptoms, then check each box that seems to fit. At the end, add up the number of times you checked each headache type and you'll have a pretty good idea what kind of headache you are suffering from. Then the next step will be to figure out what triggers your headache in the first place.

TIME OF ONSET

Recording when your headaches first began is very important. This is one of the most important differences between the various headache types.

1. At what age did your headaches begin?

If your headaches have been around for months or years and they've stayed pretty much the same, it usually means they're not due to organic disease. If your headaches have started suddenly, your chances of having an underlying illness are greatly increased, especially if they have been getting gradually worse for days to weeks. These severe, sudden-onset headaches are the most dangerous kind, unless their cause can be traced to psychological factors. Headaches that strike after a surgical procedure, childbirth, death of a loved one, or a serious economic loss, for example, may indicate an underlying depression. But when such headaches are accompanied by other symptoms, like paralysis, weakness, or strange "pinprick" sensations, it may be a warning of a serious organic disorder.

Chronic headaches fall into two general categories: tension-type headaches and vascular headaches. The latter include migraine and cluster headaches.

It's important for you to remember when your headaches first started. Migraine usually begins in adolescence or early adulthood, although it can appear in early childhood as well. Cluster headaches tend to occur for the first time in people who are in their twenties and thirties. Children also get chronic tension-type headaches, but they usually first show up during a woman's thirties and forties.

If you have recurrent headaches with symptom-free intervals, you probably suffer from vascular headaches. But some patients may suffer from a combination of migraine and tension-type headaches.

If your headaches plague you every month at about the same point in your menstrual cycle, then your headaches are probably triggered by your fluctuating menstrual hormones.

The time of day that your headaches occur can also help you identify them. Among the organic headaches, acute sinus headaches usually start gradually in the morning and increase in intensity as the day wears on. But headaches due to high blood pressure are worse upon awakening and often disappear as the day continues.

Tension-type headaches are further subdivided into anxiety headaches and depression headaches. Headaches caused by anxiety tend to strike unpredictably, at almost any time, while depression headaches establish a regular pattern, usually occurring in the early morning and early evening.

Based on the above information, which headache is most like yours?

VASCULAR HEADACHES: ❏ Migraine   ❏ Cluster

TENSION-TYPE HEADACHES: ❏ Anxiety   ❏ Depression

ORGANIC HEADACHES: ❏ Tumors or trauma

OK, how did you do? You should have made a couple of notes about when your headaches started.

LOCATION

The location of head pain is also important in determining what kind of headache you have. It is also important to assess whether the pain switches sides. Vascular headaches, like migraine or cluster headaches, are usually unilateral; in other words, the pain occurs only on one side of the head. Migraine pain frequently switches sides, either during the attack or between individual migraine attacks, but it never occurs on both sides of the head at the same time. Cluster headaches usually remain on one side but may switch sides when the next group of headaches strikes. The severe pain of a cluster headache focuses most often behind or around the eye. The eye on the affected side generally becomes red and often waters, with the eyelid drooping and the pupil constricting. The nostril on the same side may become congested. Neurologists used to think that headache pain that persisted on one side of the head always indicated the presence of an underlying, organic disease. Today we know that's simply not true.

Ninety percent of tension headaches affect both sides of the head. The headache is usually persistent and localized in one area. The pain in tension-type headache is typically described as a tightness or band of pain around the head (the "hatband effect") or as a pinched feeling in the muscles of the neck. There may be a dull aching in the forehead, and discomfort in the temples, the back of the head, or the jaw may also be involved. Often, jabs of sharp pain are felt through the dull ache. While the intensity varies throughout the day, the pain can last for weeks, months, or years.

2. Describe the location of your headache. Is it one-sided or generalized?

Based on the above information, which headache is most like yours?

VASCULAR HEADACHES: ❏ **Migraine**   ❏ **Cluster**

TENSION-TYPE HEADACHES: ❏

ORGANIC HEADACHES: ❏ **Tumors or trauma**

FREQUENCY

The most common kind of headache is the tension-type headache. It comprises 85 to 90 percent of the headache problems seen by physicians. There are two forms of tension-type headaches, episodic and chronic. The episodic type is not terribly serious and can usually be relieved by aspirin, acetaminophen (Tylenol), ibuprofen compounds, such as Advil, Nuprin and naproxen sodium (Aleve). The chronic form usually occurs on a daily basis and requires preventative therapy.

Chronic tension-type headaches occur daily or almost daily and usually continue for months, weeks, or years with no relief. Chronic tension-type headaches due to either depression or anxiety may never really go away, or they may come and go at any time of day. Activity tends to intensify the pain of tension-type headaches. Women who are afflicted with tension-type headaches due to stress may enjoy a respite from their pain during vacations. But if a woman gets headaches during periods of relaxation or the pain is worse in the morning and late afternoon, then an underlying depression may be present.

Migraines tend to vary in frequency, recurring at intervals with complete freedom from pain between attacks. Sometimes an identifiable monthly pattern can be established that links headaches with the menstrual period. This association is very important because it can be used to determine the method of treatment.

Unlike other types of headaches, cluster headaches are usually seasonal, occurring most often in spring and fall. The clusters occur together or in groups, striking one or more times daily for several weeks or months. After such onslaughts they may totally subside for reprieves that last several months or even years. Migraines may also occur more frequently in spring and fall.

3. Describe the frequency of your headache.

Based on the above information, which headache is most like yours?

VASCULAR HEADACHES: ❏ **Migraine**   ❏ **Cluster**

TENSION-TYPE HEADACHES: ❏

ORGANIC HEADACHES: ❏ **Tumors or trauma**

DURATION

If the headache is due to an organic cause like a brain tumor, it is usually constant and continuous and will progressively increase in intensity. Migraine occurs periodically and generally lasts anywhere from a few hours to a few days. Cluster headache pain can last from several minutes to almost four hours. Chronic tension-type headaches are usually constant. Episodic tension-type headaches are usually relieved by over-the-counter remedies and do not need to be addressed in this section.

4. Describe the duration of your headache.

Based on the above information, which headache is most like yours?

VASCULAR HEADACHES: ❑ **Migraine**   ❑ **Cluster**

TENSION-TYPE HEADACHES: ❑

ORGANIC HEADACHES: ❑ **Tumors or trauma**

SEVERITY OF PAIN

The pain of tension-type headache is often dull, nagging, and persistent, and tends to get worse during the day, primarily in the early morning and late afternoon. The pain of migraine may vary in intensity, but it has a pulsating or throbbing quality that sets it apart from headaches marked by a more constant type of pain. Due to the vascular nature of the headache, physical exertion increases the discomfort. Cluster headache is also throbbing, but it is frequently described as a deep, boring, severe, burning, and even unbearable pain. With an organic-type headache such as facial neuralgia the pain is shock-like, transient, or stabbing.

5. Describe the severity of your headache.

Based on the above information, which headache is most like yours?

VASCULAR HEADACHES:	❑ Migraine	❑ Cluster
TENSION-TYPE HEADACHES:	❑	
ORGANIC HEADACHES:	❑ Tumors or trauma	

WARNING SIGNS

Warning signs such as auras precede a headache in 10 to 20 percent of migraine sufferers. Auras occur anywhere from ten to thirty minutes before the acute headache attack. Although the aura is most often visual, it can involve sensory, movement, or speech impairments. It may be very minimal, such as smelling a strange odor or feeling a pins-and-needles sensation in an arm, leg, or both. The visual symptoms, however, may be more severe, causing some women to see bright stars, zigzag or wavy lines, or blind spots; some suffer loss of vision in part of their visual field.

The aura phase varies from person to person but once it develops, the aura usually remains fairly consistent. In other words, you will almost always experience the same type of aura.

6. Do you experience any auras before your headache? Describe them.

If you have auras, check Migraine.

VASCULAR HEADACHES: ❏ **Migraine**   ❏ **Cluster**

TENSION-TYPE HEADACHES: ❏

ORGANIC HEADACHES: ❏ **Tumors or trauma**

PREMONITORY SYMPTOMS OF MIGRAINE

Premonitory symptoms of migraine differ from auras because they occur twenty-four to seventy-two hours prior to the headache attack. These symptoms are usually less dramatic, but they definitely indicate a developing migraine. Sometimes they can be discerned only by a woman's spouse or close friends. Symptoms can include: anxiety, depression, excessive hunger or thirst, surges of energy, irritability, or obsessiveness.

7. *Describe any suspected premonitory symptoms before your headache.*

If you have premonitory symptoms, check Migraine.

VASCULAR HEADACHES: ❏ **Migraine**   ❏ **Cluster**

TENSION-TYPE HEADACHES: ❏ **Anxiety**   ❏ **Depression**

ORGANIC HEADACHES: ❏ **Tumors or trauma**

ASSOCIATED SYMPTOMS

Along with the head pain of migraine attacks, some women experience a host of other symptoms like sensitivity to light, loss of appetite, nausea, vomiting, and difficulty with urination. Cluster headaches may be associated with tearing eyes, drooping eyelids, nasal congestion, and facial flushing. In a patient with a brain hemorrhage, a stiff neck is one of the most prominent symptoms. Sudden loss of strength in the arms or legs associated with a headache would suggest a stroke. Ringing in the ears or double-vision on one side may indicate a brain tumor. If a headache and a seizure occur simultaneously for the first time in a patient, it also usually signifies that a serious organic disease is to blame.

8. Describe any associated symptoms.

Based on the above information, which headache is most like yours?

VASCULAR HEADACHES: ❏ Migraine   ❏ Cluster

TENSION-TYPE HEADACHES: ❏ Anxiety   ❏ Depression

ORGANIC HEADACHES: ❏ Tumors or trauma

SLEEP PATTERNS

Sleep disturbances invariably accompany tension-type headaches. Difficulty in falling asleep is indicative of anxiety. Frequent or early waking is a pattern of depression and can be an indication of depression headaches. Your physician should do a careful history to determine if stress or psychological factors may be producing your problem.

Many women will wake up at their normal time with a migraine present, but it is rare for a migraine to be severe enough to cause early waking. The stabbing pain that frequently rouses a person in the middle of the night, however, is symptomatic of a cluster-type headache. And the intensity of the pain forces them into restless activity until the attack subsides.

9. Describe any unusual sleep patterns.

Based on the above information, which headache is most like yours?

VASCULAR HEADACHES: ❏ **Migraine**   ❏ **Cluster**

TENSION-TYPE HEADACHES: ❏ **Anxiety**   ❏ **Depression**

ORGANIC HEADACHES: ❏ Tumors or trauma

OCCUPATIONAL TRIGGERS

Emotional factors, increased workloads, and stress on the job frequently initiate headaches. There are certain occupations that predispose toward headache—those that involve dealing with the public under stress or working in a migraine-triggering environment. The nitrites to which munitions workers are exposed can cause vasodilation of the cerebral vessels and mimic vascular headache. Mechanics and others who work in poorly ventilated areas can get headaches from the carbon monoxide in the atmosphere.

Tension headaches can occur as the result of poor posture after excessive reading, a long car trip, or working at a computer terminal. Chronic tension headaches are usually due to depression or anxiety.

10. Describe the suspected occupational triggers for your headache.

FAMILY HISTORY

Migraine is a familial disease, while cluster headache is not. In one study, 70 percent of female migraineurs had a mother or grandmother who suffered from migraines. Brain tumors and acute tension headaches usually do not have any family relationship. Chronic tension headaches may be seen in families as a learned behavior.

11. List all relatives who suffered from chronic headaches.

Based on the above information, which headache is most like yours?

VASCULAR HEADACHES: ❏ Migraine   ❏ Cluster

TENSION-TYPE HEADACHES: ❏ Anxiety   ❏ Depression

ORGANIC HEADACHES: ❏ Tumors or trauma

RELATIONSHIP TO MENSTRUAL CYCLE

Until the time of puberty, migraine occurs more frequently in males. With the start of menstruation, however, it becomes more common in females. During pregnancy, most migraines will disappear by the third month, only to reappear after the child has been delivered. Often migraines will wane or completely cease during menopause. The administration of hormones in the post-menopausal period frequently causes or prolongs the headache syndrome.

> **12. Do you think your headache is related to your menstrual cycle? Explain why.**

UNDERLYING MEDICAL CAUSES

Head trauma that you have experienced either recently or in the remote past can be the cause of your headache. Any blow to the head, no matter how minor, can result in a headache caused by clots developing between the covering of the brain and the brain itself. In addition, medical techniques like spinal taps or anesthesia can set off a severe headache. A history of seizures, one-sided headache, and neck stiffness can point to organic causes, such as a weak blood vessel, aneurysm, or congenital malformation of a blood vessel inside the head.

> **13. List all possible underlying medical causes.**

Based on the above information, which headache is most like yours?

VASCULAR HEADACHES: ❑ Migraine ❑ Cluster

TENSION-TYPE HEADACHES: ❑ Anxiety ❑ Depression

ORGANIC HEADACHES: ❑ Tumors or trauma

SURGICAL HISTORY

Any previous surgery or operation on the head could lead to severe headaches. Past surgery, even on a minor mole or tumor in any other part of the body, should not be ignored. A past history of tuberculosis also may have significance.

14. List all relevant surgical history.

Based on the above information, which headache is most like yours?

VASCULAR HEADACHES:	❑ Migraine	❑ Cluster
TENSION-TYPE HEADACHES:	❑ Anxiety	❑ Depression
ORGANIC HEADACHES:	❑ Tumors or trauma	

ALLERGIES

Headaches are sometimes brought on by environmental sensitivity and rarely by respiratory and food allergies. Your doctor will take an allergy history because patients, especially women, can be particularly sensitive to certain medications and these should be noted when prescribing a treatment. Do your headaches seem to follow a pattern that corresponds to meals or time spent in a certain place?

15. List all known allergies, as well as suspected food or environmental headache triggers.

Based on the above information, which headache is most like yours?

VASCULAR HEADACHES: ❑ Migraine   ❑ Cluster

TENSION-TYPE HEADACHES: ❑ Anxiety   ❑ Depression

ORGANIC HEADACHES: ❑ Tumors or trauma

PAST MEDICATIONS

Past medications can be a key to the diagnosis and treatment of your headache. If ergotamine has helped you in the past, for example, you probably suffer migraines. A history of past medications and their success or failure may yield diagnostic and therapeutic clues to the management of your headache.

If aspirin or other pain relievers have been effective in the past, then it is more likely that tension-type headaches are indicated. If your headache pain has intensified beyond the ability of over-the-counter medications to provide relief, you should consult a physician.

16. List all medications you have used in the past for your headache, and their effectiveness.

Based on the above information, which headache is most like yours?

VASCULAR HEADACHES: ❑ Migraine   ❑ Cluster

TENSION-TYPE HEADACHES: ❑ Anxiety   ❑ Depression

ORGANIC HEADACHES: ❑ Tumors or trauma

PRESENT MEDICATIONS

The current medications you are taking should also be inventoried. Birth control pills, for instance, commonly increase the frequency and severity of migraine. We also know that nitrates can activate migraine in certain susceptible people. Although indomethacin (Indocin) can help certain types of cluster and exertional headaches, it can on occasion precipitate chronic headaches. Tell your physician if you have recently begun taking any new drugs. Provide a list of medications you are currently taking, since such information may disclose that a single drug or drug combination is triggering the head pain.

> **17. List all medications you are currently taking**
> **whether for headache or not.**

Totals

All right. Now let's total up the scores from the twelve boxes entitled, "Based on the above information, which headache is most like yours?"

Based on the above information, which headache is most like yours?

VASCULAR HEADACHES: ❏ Migraine   ❏ Cluster

TENSION-TYPE HEADACHES: ❏ Anxiety   ❏ Depression

ORGANIC HEADACHES: ❏ Tumors or trauma

Most of you will come out with a pretty good idea of what type of headache you have been suffering from. If two kinds of headaches have equal or nearly equal scores, you may be plagued by coexisting migraine and tension-type headache.

Remember, once you determine what is triggering your headaches, you can almost always bring them under control. If menstrual hormones are the culprit, there is now a whole host of effective remediations. And remember, save this test and take it with you the next time you visit your doctor. It may save time and perhaps provide valuable insights into the cause of your problem.

WHEN TO CALL THE DOCTOR

One primary clue to serious disease is the sudden onset of severe and persistent headaches. This would rule out the woman with a long history of headaches that have been recurring month after month, year after year. But if a woman begins experiencing chronic headaches that increase in frequency and intensity, she should definitely be examined by a physician. Only a small proportion of headaches are caused by life-threatening maladies. In fact, it has been estimated that only 2 percent of headache sufferers have such underlying physical disorders. But because headaches caused by brain tumors can be confused with migraines and other headaches, it is important to see a physician to rule out catastrophic causes.

Headaches brought on entirely by organic causes are also called traction and inflammatory headaches. They are signs that something is physically amiss with the body or, most often, the head. They can be dangerous and require treatment by a physician.

A brain tumor is just one of several disorders with life-threatening or disabling consequences for which headache is often an initial complaint. The headache associated with a brain tumor usually strikes suddenly and grows progressively worse in a short period of time. At the onset, the brain tumor headache can be mild and easily relieved by analgesics. But it may become increasingly unbearable after changing position, such as standing up after sitting.

You should see a doctor immediately and without delay if you have a headache that comes on suddenly, especially if it feels like the worst headache you have ever had in your life. Although a headache may be the primary sign of a brain tumor, other symptoms associated with disease will usually confirm the diagnosis. If you experience loss of memory, disorientation, difficulty in making judgments, vision changes, or have seizures accompanying your headaches for the first time, you should suspect a brain tumor. Be sure to tell the doctor who examines you about any numbness or weakness in a hand, arm, or leg, and any speech or memory disorders. A brain tumor can occur at any age. If your physician suspects a brain tumor, a CT scan or an MRI will be part of the initial workup. Traction headaches can be caused by any number of other organic problems, including:

- Brain abscess

- Hematomas

- Strokes

- Aneurysms

- Meningitis or encephalitis

- Severe high blood pressure

- Normal pressure hydrocephalus

- Temporal arteritis

- Benign intercranial hypertension

All of these headache instigators can be very dangerous. For more information on these conditions, see the Glossary.

THE SIX DANGER SIGNALS

Although life-threatening headaches are rare, anyone with a headache problem, especially ones that start suddenly, should be aware of certain symptoms that indicate a need to see a doctor immediately. Such headaches can be identified by the following six danger signals:

1.   Headaches that do not fit a recognizable pattern or those that make you feel sick or "not right."

2.   Headaches that interfere with your life and prevent you from pursuing normal activities.

3.   Recurrent headaches that start after age fifty or in early childhood. In such cases a thorough investigation is imperative in order to rule out any serious underlying causes.

4.   Headaches that start suddenly and rapidly increase in frequency and intensity, when you do not have a long history of headaches. Again, a thorough general examination is indicated.

5.   Headaches accompanied by any neurological symptoms such as a temporary loss of or change in vision, motor function, or sensation.

6.   Headaches marked by any abnormal physical signs, including heart murmurs, kidney problems, or fever. In addition, stiffness of the neck may indicate an infection or inflammation of the spinal fluid.

WHERE TO GET HELP

Educating yourself and your family is essential in treating and preventing your headaches. If you have a question or want additional information or clarification, The National Headache Foundation is an organization for lay people that sponsors research in headache and serves as a resource center. You can write to the foundation for information about headaches. The foundation will also provide you with a list of physician members in your local area who are interested in the treatment of headache. The foundation is located at 5252 North Western Avenue, Chicago, Illinois 60625 (phone 800-843-2256).

2

ℋEADACHES AND YOUR ℋORMONES

The cause of headaches has been debated in medicine for 100 years. As the respected British researcher J. N. Blau put it: "Migraine, like gravity, becomes evident only by its effects. The mechanism remains mysterious. . . . "

The reason is that headaches are hard to study. Animals in a lab can't tell you about their headaches, and you can't dissect a living human brain during a migraine to see what's going on inside. We do know that many things can trigger headaches, and it frequently takes several factors combined to exceed a person's ability to resist a headache attack. This is your individual "headache threshold." It's as different in each person as each person's biochemistry is different from everyone else's.

But no matter what particular trigger is responsible for setting off your headache—be it a tension, migraine, or cluster type—we now know that many different hormones regulate the biochemical process that causes pain, including headache pain. In this sense, all headaches are essentially "hormone headaches."

After years of research, it seems that a hormonal perspective of headaches is the most accurate one. In fact, it is the basic contention of this book that hormones are one of the most important components in the biochemical chain of events that culminates in headache pain.

HORMONES, HORMONES EVERYWHERE

The greater your understanding of how your own body's biochemistry works, the better equipped you will be to take control of your pain. To do that, you need to know something about the hormones that maintain and regulate your body's incredibly complex and delicate biochemical equilibrium. Even a rudimentary knowledge of hormones is vital to an understanding of many types of headache pain.

Scientists have currently identified hundreds of hormones, but only fifty or so have been studied closely enough for scientists to be reasonably certain what their effects are in the body. New hormones are being discovered all the time; each provides us with knowledge for understanding, preventing, or aborting headaches.

The fact is we couldn't feel pain at all without hormones. Hormones induce the pain response in the first place. Hormones such as serotonin, histamine, and bradykinin are secreted by damaged cells to create a pain response in the nerve endings. Still other hormones, called prostaglandins, make the nerve endings more sensitive to these pain inducers, allowing the nerves to fire off their pain signals initially with greater ease.

As the pain travels towards the brain, it must cross nerve synapses between nerve cells. What allows that crossing? Hormones such as serotonin. These hormones are called neurotransmitters. Without these chemical messengers your body could not communicate pain messages at all.

As the pain signal nears the brain it can be stopped along the way by still other hormones. At every synapse special pain-blocking cells called interneurons can secrete natural opiate hormones called endorphins, which can block the pain signal from proceeding to the brain. Even once in the brain, other hormones called enkephalins serve the same pain-blocking function. That's how man-made opiates such as morphine and codeine work. They mimic the action of natural endorphins and enkephalins by blocking the release of the neurotransmitters necessary to carry the pain signal along.

HEADACHES AS WARNING SIGNALS

Believe it or not, your hormone-induced headaches may actually be protecting you against more damaging afflictions. Why? In the same way that the pain resulting from touching a hot stove is meant to protect your skin from a serious burn, headaches may actually be a protective mechanism designed to safeguard you from damaging agents and situations.

If you found that eating chocolate gave you migraine headaches, you would probably stop eating it, wouldn't you? A headache may be your body's way of telling you to modify certain behaviors that are harmful to you. Interestingly enough unhealthy habits like skipping meals, going without sleep, and exposure to prolonged physical or emotional stress predispose women to headaches.

WHAT ARE HORMONES?

In order to understand what role your hormones play in headache pain, it is necessary to know something about them and the manner in which they sustain the delicate, precarious chemical balance necessary for good health.

Scientists discovered hormones in 1902 when British researchers first identified digestive hormones. The word *hormone* comes from the Greek word that means to *set in motion*. And that's exactly what they do. They act as powerful and indispensable chemical messengers carried by the blood to control many of the body's functions. They initiate and regulate such body functions as digestion, growth, development, and reproduction. It is mostly hormones that determine whether you will be tall or short, fat or thin, calm or nervous, even-tempered or irritable, fast-moving or slow. If you fail to produce the proper type or amount of hormone, serious disorders—or even death—can occur.

Hormones are grouped according to their effects. *Metabolic hormones* regulate the way the body converts food into energy. For example, hormones produced in the stomach and the small intestine control the flow of digestive juices. The hormones insulin and glucagon, both secreted by the pancreas, control the amount of sugar in the blood.

Other hormones such as adrenaline (epinephrine) prepare the body for the "fight-or-flight" stress response. *Blood composition hormones* work together to ensure that levels of blood chemicals remain constant. *Growth hormones* control development during childhood and maintain the proper size and structure of certain tissues in adults. *Regulating hormones* include those that determine femininity, masculinity, and sexuality. There are even hormones that control the production of other hormones.

YOUR ENDOCRINE SYSTEM

Hormones are manufactured and secreted by endocrine glands. Endocrine glands are called "ductless" glands because

The Human Endocrine Glands

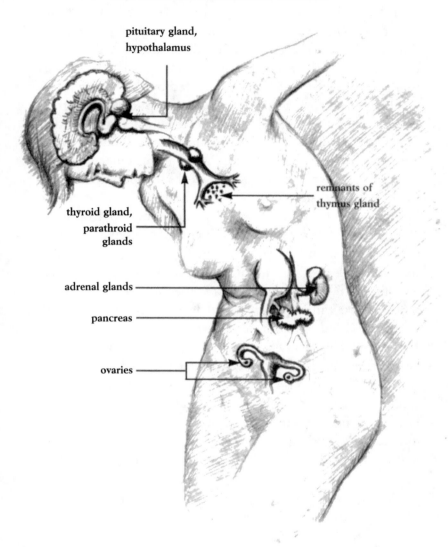

pituitary gland,
hypothalamus

remnants of
thymus gland

thyroid gland,
parathroid
glands

adrenal glands

pancreas

ovaries

they have no openings or "ducts" but secrete their respective hormones directly into your body's blood or lymph. Exocrine glands, such as sweat glands or salivary glands, on the other hand, excrete their products through ducts that lead directly to the mouth. The exocrine glands are not hormonal glands, but they may be affected by the hormones.

The endocrine glands include the pituitary, thyroid, parathyroid, thymus, adrenals, pancreas, gonads and other glandular tissues located in your intestines, kidneys, lungs, heart, and blood vessels. Together, these glands make up your endocrine system. This system works cooperatively with your nervous system to keep your body in balance and in harmony with your constantly changing environment. Working in concert, the messengers dispatched by your endocrine system and your nervous system are responsible for thousands of different automatic responses that regulate and integrate your body functions. Together, they determine whether you will respond to a headache trigger in your environment with a sensation of head pain.

In your nervous system, pain messages are conducted by electrical impulses along a network of specialized cells called neurons. The response of neurons to transmissions of these electrical messages is almost instantaneous. If you touch a hot stove, for example, the sensory nerves in your fingers immediately send out a pain message and your hand is automatically jerked away before you even have time to think about it.

In the endocrine system, on the other hand, the messengers are chemical and travel by way of the bloodstream to their receptors—specialized cells in the various organs or body tissues that are specifically programmed to receive particular hormones. These chemical messengers are the hormones produced by the pituitary/hypothalamus complex at the base of the brain, as well as other glands scattered throughout the body. Since hormones travel through the bloodstream, their responses are slower than neural reactions. Because only tiny amounts of hormones circulate in the blood, the hormones themselves must be incredibly efficient and their receptor sites must be amazingly sensitive in order to achieve their desired effects.

Just try to visualize it for a moment. As a hormone travels through your blood, it seeks out receptor sites that are specifically programmed to receive it. Since protein hormones like insulin are too large to enter cells themselves, their receptor sites lie on the outside of their target cells. As soon as a protein hormone connects with its receptor site, the receptor relays the hormone's message inside the target cell to the part that is designed to respond to the hormone. But in order to do this other reactions must be involved. The hormone must activate an enzyme called adenylcyclase, located in the cell membrane. Once activated this enzyme forms a second messenger, or hormone "mediator," called cyclic AMP, which actually carries out the hormonal action.

Unlike insulin, however, other hormones are small enough to cross their target cell's membrane and don't need to bind to a receptor site on the cell's surface. Steroid hormones, for example, seek out and attach to a receptor site within the target cell itself. Once that happens the hormone and receptor combine to form a smaller molecule that actually enters the inner sanctum of the cell nucleus, where it goes directly to its own encoded portion of DNA. This activates specific genes to form the messenger RNA that carries out the hormone's original purpose. Since RNA and DNA carry the genetic information that causes fluctuations in hormones (and can lead to menstrual headaches), understanding the role of these hormones and their secondary messengers should help us find ways to interrupt the hormonal process-es that trigger headaches.

Like cyclic AMP, substances called prostaglandins act as secondary messengers also, carrying out hormonal commands and performing many hormone-directed functions. Cyclic AMP and prostaglandins both perform many different func-tions, depending on which tissues make them and the par-ticular hormones that order them around.

In the uterus, for example, prostaglandins stimulate mus-cle contractions and are thought to initiate labor when a woman is ready to give birth. Likewise, during menstruation prostaglandins cause uterine contractions. And as you might have guessed, an overproduction of prostaglandins causes the painful menstrual cramps that plague so many women. It is no coincidence that the monthly headaches that tend to afflict women around the time of their periods occur when prostaglandin production is high. Indeed, prostaglandins are thought to play a central role in many kinds of headache pain.

In fact, almost all of the major endocrine glands secrete hormones that have been implicated in head pain. These include the pituitary, thyroid, parathyroid, adrenals, pan-creas, and gonads. Different headache triggers appear to spark head pain because they set in motion a chain of bio-chemical events in which hormones play a major role. To understand what that role is, it is necessary, of course, to know something about the different hormones and the glands that manufacture and secrete them.

THE PITUITARY

Located deep inside your head, your pituitary gland is situ-ated behind the nasal cavities and just below the hypothala-mus at the base of the brain. The hypothalamus is part of the forebrain, or diencephalon, and links the thinking part of the brain with the pituitary gland. The hypothalamus regulates many endocrine functions, especially through its control of the pituitary gland. The pituitary gland itself produces many of the hormones that control other glands; for this reason it is often called the body's master gland. If one takes into account the pituitary's wide variety of hormones and functions, it is only to be expected that disorders of the hypothalamus and pituitary can have a profound effect on the absence or presence of chronic headaches.

The pituitary is divided into two parts, or lobes. The back part, or posterior lobe, actually connects the gland to the hypothalamus and is more nerve-like in makeup, while the front part, or anterior lobe, is made up of glandular tissue. Hormones manufactured in the pituitary's anterior lobe are mostly trophic, meaning that they stimulate other glands or organs to go into action. One group of trophic hormones, known as gonadotrophins, have been implicated in headache attacks. In a woman, these gonadotrophins include FSH (follicle-stimulating hormone), which prompts the ovaries to ripen an egg each month, and LH (luteinizing hormone), which stimulates the ovarian follicle to release a ripened egg (see chapter 3).

Other pituitary hormones that have been linked to headache include ACTH (adrenal-cortex-stimulating hormone), which stimulates the adrenal glands to produce their hormones, TSH (thyroid-stimulating hormone), which stimulates the thyroid gland to produce its hormones, and vasopressin, which controls the muscle tone of blood vessels. Vasopressin also acts as an antidiuretic hormone that helps the kidneys conserve water and maintain the body's fluid balance.

Prolactin is another pituitary hormone that has been implicated in the biochemical dysfunction that causes headaches. Prolactin initiates and maintains the production of breast milk in nursing mothers. It also performs other more mysterious metabolic duties. For instance, we know that during migraine attacks there is a disturbance of the body's prolactin-regulating systems. In fact, it appears that a woman's prolactin secreting mechanism becomes hyperactive during a migraine attack. Studies now show that some of the major migraine triggers—stress, exercise, and the use of oral contraceptives—all produce higher-than-normal levels of prolactin in the blood. Interestingly enough, some anti-migraine drugs (ergot alkaloids and clonidine) have a pro-lactin suppressing effect, lending support to the idea that high prolactin levels are a causative factor in migraine.

THE THYROID

Traveling downward from your pituitary, the next major endocrine gland you'll come across is your thyroid. Lying over your windpipe, just beneath your larynx, it is a butter-fly-shaped structure that normally weighs only an ounce or less. Despite its small size, its hormones are necessary to the proper function of nearly every organ and system in your body. And like the pituitary, the hormones your thyroid gland secretes are involved in the biochemical process that causes head pain.

Three such hormones are triiodothyronine and thyrox-ine, which control metabolism by increasing the oxygen con-sumption of cells, and calcitonin, which is instrumental in calcium metabolism. When too much or too little of these hormones are secreted by the thyroid gland, chronic headaches may result. Too much thyroid hormone causes a condition called hyperthyroidism that speeds up the metab-olism. It is characterized by a rapid heartbeat, a jittery, ner-vous irritability, muscle weakness, fatigue, and weight loss.

Excessive sweating and an intolerance to heat can also signal an overactive thyroid gland.

An underactive thyroid gland, on the other hand, slows almost all body processes. The skin, fingernails, and hair become dry and brittle due to a slowdown in their growth. Intestinal activity grows more sluggish also, resulting in constipation. Other symptoms include headache, a slow heart rate, fatigue, lethargy, intolerance to cold, puffiness of the legs and ankles from accumulation of body fluids, muscular soreness, and leg cramps.

The serious health problems that can result from an overactive or underactive thyroid illustrate why it is so important to seek medical help from a headache specialist if you are plagued by chronic headaches. Such headaches are sometimes a symptom of a deeper underlying health problem that needs to be addressed.

THE PARATHYROID

On the back and side of each thyroid lobe are small, disk-shaped nodules that make up your parathyroid gland. Most people have four of these tiny glands, but the number can vary. The glands secrete a parathyroid hormone that acts to raise the level of calcium circulating in the bloodstream; meanwhile, calcitonin (produced by the thyroid) acts to lower those levels. If the parathyroid malfunctions, calcium levels in the blood may fall too low. Calcium in the blood is essential for your muscles and nerves to work properly.

THE THYMUS

Lying behind the sternum, or breastbone, is the thymus gland. Probably the strangest endocrine gland in the human body, its function is not yet fully understood. Researchers tell us that this mysterious gland is made up mostly of lymphoid tissue and that it is instrumental in the production of cells that are essential to the immune system.

Babies are born with a large thymus gland, which continues to grow until puberty. After that it begins to shrink, which is why it is very small in older people. Chinese medicine believes the thymus to be the seat of the body's ability to fend off disease and aging. Practitioners of an ancient Chinese healing art known as Qigong (pronounced Cheekong) have special exercises devoted to opening up the thymus gland to perpetuate its functioning.

THE PANCREAS

Moving down the body from the parathyroid and thymus, the next major endocrine gland that plays a role in headache pain is the pancreas. It is a long, narrow organ that lies across most of the upper abdomen, just below the breasts. Although the pancreas also acts as an exocrine gland, manufacturing and secreting digestive enzymes that travel through pancreatic ducts to the small intestine to aid digestion, it is the hormonal secretions of the gland that play a role in headache pain.

This vital gland produces the hormones insulin, glucagon, and somatostatin, which ensure that your body maintains just the right levels of blood sugar, or glucose, to operate properly. Just as gasoline is the fuel that powers your car, glucose is the fuel that runs your body. Without it the cells throughout your body would literally starve to death. It is easy to see how such important hormones could initiate or aggravate the biochemical processes that cause headache. Skipping meals, for example, frequently triggers headaches because the practice causes blood sugar levels to fall. This type of low blood sugar, or hypoglycemia, is called "reactive" hypoglycemia because it occurs in reaction to skipping meals.

You can counteract the insulin gush that follows high-carbohydrate meals by adding protein and fat to your breakfast or by eating a snack in the midmorning and mid-afternoon to take care of the large amount of insulin pro-duced by a sugary breakfast or a high-carbohydrate lunch.

Keep in mind that drinking alcoholic beverages can also cause hypoglycemia and the headaches that go along with it. But unlike diet-related hypoglycemia, alcohol lowers blood sugar by interfering with the body's ability to make glucose. Drinking on an empty stomach or several hours before eat-ing is particularly harmful.

THE ADRENALS

Your adrenal glands are a pair of triangular-shaped glands that sit on top of your kidneys. Each of these glands is divid-ed into two parts with an inner section called the medulla and an outer layer called the cortex. Each part produces completely different hormones.

The adrenal medulla makes a group of hormones called catecholamines, which include the stress hormones adrena-line (sometimes known as epinephrine), and noradrenaline (or norepinephrine). Another catecholamine hormone-like substance, dopamine, is thought to vary with some of the blood vessel changes that occur during migraines.

The catecholamine hormones play an important role in the fight-or-flight response. The production of adrenaline and noradrenaline is boosted the instant your body perceives danger. Your body reacts the same way to stress, low blood sugar, exposure to cold, an oxygen shortage, lowered blood pressure, and many other stressful situations. In fact, any stressful situation, from an angry boss to a crying infant, can trigger the increased output of these adrenal hormones.

The adrenal cortex manufactures a whole group of hormones referred to as steroids. These, in turn, are divided into three categories according to their function in the body. The *mineralocorticoids* control the body's fluid balance by regulating the kidney's reabsorption of sodium and potassium. The *glucocorticoids* help regulate the metabolism of glucose (blood sugar) and other nutrients, maintain blood pressure, and enable the body to respond to physical stress. The *sex hormones (androgens and estrogens)* are responsible for male and female characteristics.

One of the major *mineralocorticoids*, aldosterone, helps the kidneys conserve sodium and so maintains the body's fluid balance. An overproduction of this adrenal hormone leads to abnormally high sodium levels in the blood, a condition that may result in high blood pressure and potassium deficiency, which may lead, in turn, to muscular weakness, cramps, and tension headaches.

The most plentiful of the *glucocorticoids* are cortisol and corticosterone. The liver metabolizes cortisol into cortisone, a steroid that is commonly used to treat allergic conditions like asthma, and inflammatory disorders like arthritis.

Cortisol has an anti-insulin effect that is vital to the conversion of protein and fats into glucose—the body's major fuel. The adrenal glands react to any stress or injury to the body by increasing cortisol production, which increases blood sugar levels to increase your energy level. It is cortisol's job to counter the harmful effects of injury or infection. During this fight-or-flight response, the brain signals the pituitary gland to manufacture the hormone ACTH, which tells the adrenals to secrete extra cortisol and cate-cholamines.

Both of these hormones have similar functions and produce the familiar stress-related symptoms of more rapid and more forceful heartbeat. The improved blood circulation that results promotes alertness. It also speeds up metabolism by breaking down fats more quickly than usual, thus providing extra energy. Noradrenaline raises blood pressure by constricting or narrowing blood vessels. Adrenaline constricts some blood vessels but, more important, opens up others in the muscles and the liver. As a result, more blood is carried to the muscles to endow you with the extra strength needed to escape danger.

SEX HORMONES

The *sex hormones* consist of androgens and estrogens. Although both men's and women's bodies produce androgen, androgen levels in men are far higher. It is from androgen that men get their "maleness" and from the estrogen hormones that women get their "femaleness." But strangely enough it is actually the androgens, or male hormones, secreted by a woman's adrenal glands that are responsible for a woman's libido, or sex drive. Of course androgens also control male libido, but in men, the testes make most of this sex hormone.

Not until fairly recently did researchers fully realize just how influential your ovaries may be in causing headache pain. Studies indicate that this pair of almond-sized glands, nestled deep in a woman's pelvis, hold the key to understanding the phenomenon of "menstrual headaches." Medical science now has confirmed what millions of women had long suspected—that the same hormones that controlled their menstrual cycle were also responsible for their monthly headaches.

Obviously, a woman's "sex hormones" are vital to her health. Yet they can also be responsible for the agonizing pain of chronic headaches. These headaches subject women to a kind of torture that ranges from unpleasant to unbearably excruciating. The hormones that cause women's menstrual headaches are mainly those that control the menstrual period: estrogen, progesterone, luteinizing hormone (LH), luteotropin (LTH), and follicle stimulating hormone (FSH).

Before puberty, for example, the incidence of migraine is equal for boys and girls, but after puberty, migraine incidence in women jumps to four-to-eight times that of men. Puberty usually occurs in women in the early teenage years, ages eleven to fifteen. At this time, the hypothalamus sends a hormonal message to the pituitary to start secreting the hormones FSH and LH.

Under the influence of the increased levels of FSH and LH, the ovaries grow and begin to secrete large amounts of the female sex hormones estrogen and progesterone. Estrogens cause the female sex organs to develop fully. They also stimulate the development of secondary female characteristics, such as full breasts and wide hips.

Most women begin getting their headaches in their teenage years at the start of their menstrual cycle. As adults the vast majority of women say that their headaches begin near the first day of menstruation.

But it's not only higher levels of the female hormones, estrogen and progesterone, that induce menstrual headaches. Any sudden changes in the levels of these hormones also seem to trigger headaches. During the premenstrual phase, for example, just before the menstrual flow begins, the ovarian hormones estrogen and progesterone drop dramatically. The infamous premenstrual syndrome and the headaches that come with it are clearly caused by such hormonal fluctuations.

HISTAMINE

Histamine is a hormone produced by tissues throughout the body. The digestive system also converts many food ingredients into histamine. Histamine acts to increase stomach acid and dilate capillaries. The body releases histamine when the immune system responds to an allergy-provoking substance. Histamine may be one of the hormones implicated in the dilation of the blood vessels causing post-migraine and cluster headaches. It's possible that the nausea associated with migraine may stem from the action of histamine.

3

*H*ORMONES AND THE *M*ENSTRUAL *C*YCLE

CYCLE OF PAIN—A CASE HISTORY

Anne Caraher, a successful corporate attorney, was thirty-seven when she first came to see me and related her twenty-year history of chronic monthly headaches. Her life was a cycle of pain that revolved around the agonizing migraines and menstrual cramps that peaked over a several-day period each month. She was desperate to stop the headaches.

Besides her hectic legal practice, Anne was a single mother, raising two grade-school children. Anne's life had been overshadowed by the one to three days each month when she was "crippled" with a migraine headache. She was forced to reschedule appointments and cancel activities with her children.

Throughout college and law school, the monthly headaches had become as much of a routine as midterms and finals. She scheduled her life around the few days each month that she had to stay in bed. Studying was especially difficult during her migraine attacks because bright lights and her intense nausea bothered her as long as the headaches lingered. She was forced to read wearing sunglasses, with a bucket nearby in case she had to vomit.

Anne's family doctor had prescribed an ergot suppository to use at the first sign of an oncoming migraine since the vomiting that accompanied her attacks made it impossible to swallow any medications. The suppositories sometimes helped if she didn't wake up with a headache that was already under way. To make matters worse, the pain of Anne's headaches was aggravated by severe menstrual cramping.

Despite her monthly battles with pain, Anne passed the Illinois bar exam. A few months later she married one of her law school classmates and settled down in a north shore Chicago suburb. Her first child was born just two years later, and during the pregnancy the headaches disappeared. For the first time in ten years, Anne didn't have to schedule her life around her excruciating headaches. For almost a year, Anne was able to lead a normal, pain-free life.

She hoped that the headaches had disappeared forever. But when her son, Timmy, was four months old, her monthly bouts of pain returned. Her periods had started again, and Anne knew that the old routine she dreaded so much was back. Raising a baby and working four days a week was taking its toll, and the migraine attacks added tremendously to her stress. Anne's headaches stopped again briefly when she became pregnant with her second child. But her reprieve was short-lived. When Anne stopped nursing her baby daughter, she was hit by an agonizing, three-day headache.

Years later, after struggling through a bitter divorce and returning to a full-time legal practice, Anne finally came to me for help. It has now been a year since she started treatment. Anne is overjoyed that during that time she has suffered only one moderate migraine, which lasted just a few hours. She and her children are delighted that several days each month have been "returned" to them. Anne also knows that if her daughter experiences painful menstrual headaches, help is available.

Anne's headaches were clearly being triggered by her menstrual hormones. By that I mean that they were obviously linked to the hormonal changes her body went through each month during her menstrual cycle. Headaches generated by fluctuating menstrual hormones strike women of all ages, some afflicting teenagers just entering puberty, others hitting women just entering menopause.

Although it is now a well-established fact that menstrual-related hormones can initiate the agonizing headaches that plague so many women, menstrual hormones are not the actual *cause* of the pain. They are just one of the many triggers that ignite headache pain.

Like Anne, most women are all too familiar with the symptoms that precede menstruation. Depression, irritability, abdominal bloating, and fatigue often plague women just before and during their periods. Worse still, such complaints are frequently compounded by menstrual headaches that return with painful regularity each month. These headaches may strike either as full-blown migraines or less severe tension-type headaches. But whichever form they assume, menstrual headaches are a painful ordeal for the ten million American women afflicted with them.

WHAT IS MENSTRUAL MIGRAINE?

Menstrual migraines are migraines that occur in a predictable monthly pattern before, during, or immediately after a woman's period, or during ovulation. They typically begin as a one-sided, throbbing headache accompanied by nausea, vomiting, or sensitivity to bright lights and sounds. Many women experience the vision changes that precede a classic migraine attack.

In its classic form, migraine hits on the side opposite the side on which the aura is seen, often just behind the eyebrow. In non-classic migraine the pain may turn up on either side of the head. Indeed, sometimes it occurs first on one side, later on the other side. The pain is severe—different from the very sharp pain of a cluster headache—and throbbing. If the headache lasts long enough, the pain becomes constant.

Why don't all women suffer menstrual migraines? Because susceptibility to migraines appears to be an inherited trait. Some women are genetically predisposed to the headaches. These women also have blood platelets that aggregate, or clump, more readily than normal. In addition, there appears to be a genetic vulnerability to headaches triggered by fluctuating menstrual hormones in certain women.

Researchers first discovered the connection between menstruation and headache in the 1960s. They found that 70 percent of women who suffer from migraine attacks get their headaches around the time of their periods. For years doctors could only speculate about the cause of these menstrual headaches. Now it is becoming increasingly clear that the vast majority of them are caused by the hormonal fluctuations that regulate the menstrual cycle itself. Equipped with this new understanding, doctors can now provide relief to more than 80 percent of the women who suffer severe, recurrent, menstrual headaches.

Women with recurrent menstrual headaches have the

advantage of knowing when to expect the unwelcome arrival of their next headache. They can arm themselves in advance with the very latest therapies from the medical world's anti-headache arsenal.

PHASES OF THE MENSTRUAL CYCLE

A woman's body undergoes marked physical changes during the four distinct stages of the menstrual cycle. What we call menstruation is actually the climax of these phases. Since menstrual headaches are triggered by shifting levels of the five basic hormones involved in menstruation, it is helpful to learn something about each phase.

After puberty women must journey through these phases every month of their lives until they reach menopause. Knowing more about these menstrual stages better equips women to cope with the physiological symptoms of each phase and enables them to feel more in control of their bodies.

Post-Menstrual Phase (Fifth to Ninth Day)

After menstrual bleeding stops, the next four or five days of a woman's cycle constitute the resting, or post-menstrual, phase. During this time, the lining of the uterus is very thin because most of it has been shed during menstruation. The five basic menstrual hormones—estrogen, progesterone, LH, LTH, and FSH—have ebbed to their lowest levels. Women with menstrual headaches usually feel best during this part of their monthly cycle. Most are symptom free and enjoy a sense of physical and emotional well-being.

The hormonal action starts again when the pituitary gland begins to secrete a substance known as follicle stimulating hormone (FSH). Inside a woman's ovary, high levels of

FSH LEVELS

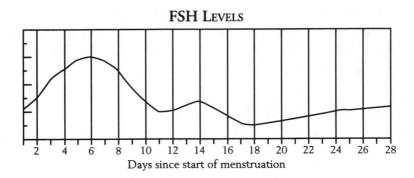

Days since start of menstruation

this hormone cause an egg to begin ripening in a tiny sac called a follicle. Incredibly, although each ovary contains as many as 400,000 potential egg cells, only one egg usually matures during each menstrual cycle. Women who are being treated for infertility are often given too much FSH, causing multiple eggs to mature and resulting in multiple births.

Normally, FSH levels usually peak around the seventh day after menstruation begins. By the end of this phase, other hormones start to control the menstrual cycle. The ovaries begin producing estrogen, which makes the lining of the uterus start to thicken.

ESTROGEN LEVELS

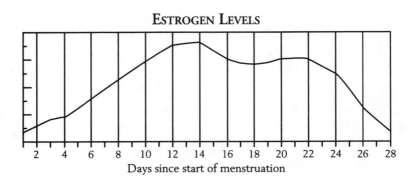

Days since start of menstruation

Proliferative Phase (Ninth to Fourteenth Day)

Most women who suffer from menstrual headaches are still symptom-free from the ninth or tenth day to the fourteenth day of their menstrual cycle. During this time, the lining of the uterus thickens rapidly, increasing sixfold to eightfold.

Within the ovary, an egg is maturing inside its protective sac until it too starts manufacturing estrogen. As FSH levels drop, estrogen levels rise dramatically. About the ninth day, the pituitary gland begins to secrete a hormone called the luteinizing hormone (LH).

LH LEVELS

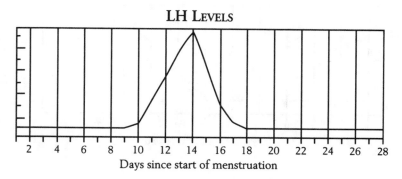

Days since start of menstruation

Levels of this hormone increase sharply over the course of several days until it finally causes the sac encasing the egg to break around the fourteenth day. The mature egg is released, and ovulation begins.

Premenstrual Phase (Fourteenth to Twenty-eighth Day)

Ovulation ushers in the premenstrual phase of a woman's cycle when many women begin experiencing the headaches and other troubling symptoms that characterize this notorious part of the menstrual cycle.

As the mature egg travels down the fallopian tube toward the uterus, hormone levels of LH drop rapidly, and

LTH LEVELS

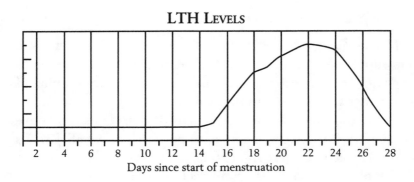

Days since start of menstruation

PROGESTERONE LEVELS

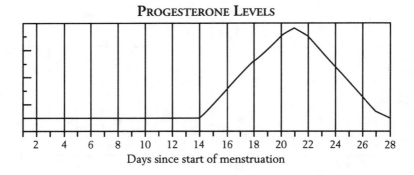

Days since start of menstruation

estrogen levels begin to dip also. The pituitary gland secretes still another hormone, luteotropin (LTH), which in turn stimulates the ovaries to produce progesterone. Progesterone helps prepare the lining of the uterus to receive and nurture the egg if it is fertilized by male sperm.

Together with estrogen, the progesterone prompts the cells of the uterine lining to change shape and expand. The blood supply increases as new blood vessels rapidly develop within the thickened lining of the uterus, providing a nourishing bed for a fertilized egg. Since the egg can survive only for one day, a woman will be fertile and able to conceive a child only during this brief, twenty-four hour period.

Menstrual Phase (First to Fifth Day)

If the egg is not fertilized, the production of estrogen and progesterone stops around the twenty-fifth day of the cycle, and the lining of the uterus starts to break down. The pituitary gland begins producing oxytocin, the hormone that causes the uterus to contract. These contractions produce the painful cramps so often associated with menstruation as countless small blood vessels and cells rupture, discharging small fragments of the uterine lining. This discharge, lasting from the first to the fifth day of the cycle, constitutes the menstrual flow.

MENSTRUAL HEADACHES

It is becoming clear that rapid shifts in the levels of menstrual-related hormones, particularly progesterone and estrogen, play a significant role in menstrual headaches. Headache activity increases, for example, when estrogen levels are in flux, either rising or falling, or when there is a change in the estrogen-to-progesterone ratio. Researchers are trying to determine if softening or buffering these dramatic swings in hormone concentrations can reduce migraine incidence.

In one study, the hormonal changes responsible for recurrent menstrual migraine were studied in eight women who suffered from the headaches. As expected, progesterone and estrogen levels fell simultaneously among all the women during the premenstrual phase of their menstrual cycles. And in all cases migraine began either during or at the end of their premenstrual hormone withdrawal phase, as levels of estrogen and progesterone declined.

When the women were given supplementary progesterone injections to forestall falling levels of the hormone, two of the women benefited. One avoided migraine altogether, while the other experienced only a mild half-hour headache instead of her usual one-to-two-day killer migraine with its accompanying nausea and visual disturbances.

The effects of estrogen supplementation, however, were far more pronounced. In all eight of the women, migraine was completely averted until several days after the estrogen injection was given. But as soon as estrogen levels had fallen to normal premenstrual levels, the typical migraines struck as expected.

In the same study, two women who had stopped having headaches when they ceased menstruating during menopause developed migraines several days after receiving an estrogen injection. Their migraines corresponded to declining estrogen levels and "estrogen withdrawal" following the estrogen "high" generated by their estrogen injections a few days before.

As a result of these findings another study was carried out in which estrogen implants were used in five women with menstrual migraines in an attempt to maintain stable estrogen levels throughout the menstrual cycle. It was hoped that this would prevent the normal premenstrual estrogen withdrawal that causes migraine in susceptible women and in addition would avoid the "rebound" migraines that struck several days after the estrogen injections wore off. None of the women in this study, however, experienced any reduction in their headache symptoms. The reason? It is impossible to enhance the body's natural ability or evenness or to achieve truly stable estrogen levels in the blood with estrogen implants, injections, or supplements.

Interestingly enough, the direct connection between too much estrogen and migraine also has been well established. Women with migraine have higher than average levels of estrogen to begin with. It appears that these higher estrogen levels precede an abnormally precipitous drop in estrogen levels during the premenstrual phase. This estrogen "crash" seems to "prime" cranial blood vessels, making them more susceptible to the vasoconstrictor serotonin that triggers headaches. Add still more estrogen in the form of birth control pills, and you would expect such women to experience more migraines. Up to 49 percent of them do.

In fact, among women who never suffered menstrual headaches before they began using oral contraceptives, 10 percent started getting the headaches after they began taking the Pill. Headache is one of the most common side effects of oral contraceptive use. It has been well documented that the use of birth control pills and other estrogen compounds greatly increases the frequency, duration, severity, and complications of migraine headache. One study, conducted at a migraine headache clinic in England, found that 25 percent of women were hit with more severe or more frequent migraine attacks when they started using birth control pills.

Not surprisingly, women on the Pill also get more migraines at the midpoint of their cycle, when their own natural estrogen levels are rising most sharply. The sudden shift of estrogen from low levels preceding ovulation to the highest levels at the time of ovulation, is exacerbated by the extra estrogen in òral contraceptives. Among women sensitive to these shifts, any abrupt change in estrogen levels whether it be from low to high levels or from high to low levels appears to trigger menstrual migraine.

Why? Although the connection between shifting hormones and menstrual headaches is now well established, the exact chemical reactions involved are not. Research is focusing on abnormal platelet aggregation, which causes the release of serotonin from the platelets. This sets off a chemical chain reaction resulting in not only constriction of the blood vessels deep inside the brain but also the production of pain-causing prostaglandins.

Dramatic fluctuations in estrogen levels tend to boost prostaglandin levels in susceptible women. Although prostaglandins are crucial to an infinite array of normal body functions, these hormone-like messenger chemicals also have been identified as one of the causative factors in many of the body's pain-producing conditions, including menstrual headaches. Found in most of the body's cells, they are manufactured from polyunsaturated, essential fatty acids released from cell membranes.

Prostaglandin production in the body is a three-step process. First, the vegetables and meat we eat every day are converted to an essential fatty acid called arachidonic acid. The presence of arachidonic acid poses no problems for a woman predisposed to menstrual headaches until her hormones begin fluctuating.

When hormones begin to fluctuate, arachidonic acid converts into the unstable chemicals thromboxane and prostacyclin. During the preliminary stage of a headache, thromboxane constricts the brain's blood vessels. At the same time, shifting hormone levels cause blood platelets to begin to clump and release serotonin, another powerful constrictor. This combination causes the first stage, the aura phase of a migraine attack.

Sensing too much constriction of the blood vessels within the brain, other hormones signal the platelets to stop serotonin secretion. Not long after, the other unstable product of arachidonic acid, prostacyclin, gets in on the action and causes the arteries to dilate. Because there is already a lack of serotonin in the bloodstream, the arteries become extremely dilated.

Finally, thromboxane and prostacycalin cause cells to excrete prostaglandin hormones. Prostaglandin increases the perception of pain. More important, it causes the already dilated blood vessel walls to become inflamed, leading to the throbbing pain a migraine sufferer experiences.

If the finger of blame can be put on a single chemical substance as the main cause of migraines, it may well be prostaglandins. Researchers have shown that injections of prostaglandins all by themselves can generate the classic symptoms of migraine, complete with its visual warning signs.

Interestingly enough, the way aspirin works is to interrupt the chain of events leading from breakdown of arachidonic acid to the secretion of prostaglandin hormones. Aspirin and other nonsteroidal anti-inflammatory drugs (NSAIDs) can inhibit prostaglandin activity and actually prevent or in some cases eradicate active migraine attacks.

NATURAL PAINKILLERS

Normally the body prevents or reduces headache pain with a naturally occurring group of pain-relieving hormones, called endogenous opioids. One of these endogenous opioids is known as beta-endorphin (β-EP). Recent studies have shown that migraine patients have less of this β-EP flowing through their central nervous system.

PMS HEADACHES

Another kind of menstrual headache is referred to as PMS headache. The time it strikes, before menses begins each month, and the host of non-headache symptoms that accompany this kind of headache set it apart from "normal" menstrual headaches.

Women who get headaches during the premenstrual period (the fourteenth to the twenty-eighth day of their cycle) usually suffer from tension-type headaches or a combination of migraine and tension-type headaches. As though these headaches weren't bad enough, the discomfort of PMS headaches is compounded by physical, emotional, and behavioral changes that tend to start after ovulation, and last for one to fourteen days, before disappearing twenty-four to forty-eight hours before menstruation begins.

Abnormally low levels of the hormone serotonin may cause the dilation of blood vessels during tension-type headaches associated with PMS just as it does in the second, or headache, phase of a migraine attack. As with migraines, estrogen and progesterone fluctuations appear to trigger this biochemical response among women whose tension-type headaches are linked to their menstrual cycle.

Women with PMS headaches typically endure headache pain accompanied by fatigue, acne, joint pain, decreased urination, constipation, and lack of coordination. Increased appetite is not unusual, and women may notice a craving for sugar, chocolate, salt, or alcohol. In really severe cases women complain of fear, panic attacks, decreased sexual desire, impaired judgment or memory, difficulty concentrating, sensitivity to rejection, and paranoia, combined with a desire to be alone.

The good news is that these symptoms usually disappear when menstruation begins. The bad news is that the discomfort associated with PMS headaches is often so severe that it is nearly impossible for women with this kind of head pain to function normally. Despite this severity, most women with premenstrual headaches try to treat themselves.

Such women usually rely on rest and over-the-counter (OTC) NSAIDs like aspirin, acetaminophen, and ibuprofen to cope with their premenstrual headache pain. Many women also try to relieve their PMS headaches with non-prescription drugs like Midol PMS or Premsyn PMS, which contain acetaminophen, a diuretic, and an antihistamine. But if her symptoms are severe, a woman may get very little relief from these OTC products.

Although the physical causes of the wide range of symptoms associated with PMS headache are not clearly understood, the dramatic rise and fall of estrogen, progesterone, and the pituitary hormone luteotropin during the premenstrual phase is believed to trigger the head pain and depression associated with PMS headaches.

Treating PMS headaches with prostaglandin inhibitors has proven remarkably helpful since high levels of prostaglandins have been found to play the same role in PMS headaches that they do in menstrual headaches. Women treated with prostaglandin inhibitor drugs such as NSAIDs reported fewer PMS headaches, fewer aches and pains, and fewer emotional symptoms involving mood swings, pessimism, and irritability. Antidepressants also have been used to banish PMS headaches.

In really severe cases, some physicians will prescribe anovulation therapy as another treatment option. The term anovulation therapy refers to treatment aimed at suppressing ovulation, menstruation, and cyclic changes with the help of special hormones. Birth control pills are commonly used in this kind of therapy. This therapy should not be used for migraine sufferers because of the previously discussed effects of the Pill on migraines.

A woman whose PMS headaches are set off by rapidly declining estrogen and progesterone levels during the premenstrual phase, for example, would benefit from the additional progesterone and estrogen provided by oral contraceptives since they would act to stabilize her hormonal balance. Indeed, such women have found that treating their PMS with estrogen-progestin drug combinations, or oral contraceptives that contain only progestin (a synthetic form of progesterone), are sometimes effective.

Researchers have discovered that many untreatable cases of premenstrual syndrome (PMS), including the headaches it causes, could be alleviated by giving supplemental doses of progesterone to women. According to one researcher, more than 90 percent of patients have found relief from PMS symptoms with progesterone.

The fact that oral contraceptives worsen PMS headaches in some women and help prevent them in others suggests that each woman has her own individual hormone profile. A woman whose PMS headaches are linked to excessively high estrogen and progesterone levels, as is characteristic of menstrual sufferers, would experience a worsening of her headache and other PMS symptoms by taking the Pill.

Another drug that would be useful to treat PMS headache and other menstrual symptoms is depo-medroxy progesterone acetate (Depo-Provera). It has been used by women throughout the world as a contraceptive. This drug suppresses ovulation and menstruation, essentially producing a premature, reversible menopause. It can prove beneficial for women who are unresponsive to other forms of PMS headache treatment, but it requires careful monitoring.

SUMMARY SHEET: MENSTRUAL AND PMS HEADACHES

Symptoms: Physical fatigue, headache, abdominal bloating, breast tenderness and swelling, acne, joint pain, decreased urination, constipation, and uncoordination, emotional depression, anxiety, hostility, and anger. Other symptoms include sensitivity to rejection, desire to be alone, panic attacks, fear, decreased sexual desire, sensitivity to noise,

light, and touch, confusion, decreased ability to concentrate, impaired judgment and memory, tendency to be verbally critical of others, increased appetite, and craving for sugar, chocolate, salt, or alcohol. Some women may experience marked psychological reactions to other symptoms and suffer from feelings of guilt, shame, nonassertiveness, worthlessness, decreased self-esteem and self-confidence, and a distorted and negative body image and hopelessness.

Unique Symptoms: These headaches differ from other headaches in that they occur at regular times during the monthly menstrual cycle.

Typical Duration and Severity: One to fourteen days of symptoms during premenstrual phase. Symptoms usually disappear twenty-four to forty-eight hours after the onset of the menstrual flow. Severity of symptoms is variable; many women with severe or prolonged symptoms may have marked psychological reactions.

Treatment Strategies: NSAIDs and over-the-counter medications may relieve some symptoms. For prolonged headaches, oral contraceptives, prostaglandin inhibitors, and progesterone have been found to be effective. In severe cases, antidepressants, diuretics; progesterone; prostaglandin inhibitors; oral contraceptives; depo-medroxyprogesterone (Depo-Provera), progesterone supplements.

Effective Self-Treatments: Daily program of exercise; biofeedback. Please see chapter 10 for a full discussion of self-treatments.

When to See Your Doctor: You should consult a physician when PMS symptoms seriously affect your daily life.

4

*M*IGRAINE

Zoe Rosencrantz was a twenty-seven-year-old bookkeeper who had it all. Slim and vivacious, she was known for her quick laugh and keen wit. Although Zoe was a conscientious worker, she was also a great socializer who lived for weekends and vacations. On Fridays and Saturdays she spent her evenings at parties or dance clubs. During the summer she worked on her tan at Oak Street Beach and organized beach volleyball games. Winter weekends would find her skiing in northern Michigan, and long holidays signaled her departure to Colorado. Her parents worried she would never settle down, while Zoe worried about the day she would *have* to slow down her fast-paced, fun-filled lifestyle.

But for one week each month, Zoe was a different person. About six days before her period she would succumb to inexplicable crying jags and uncontrollable anxiety. The terrible migraines that followed were even worse. She always knew when the migraines were about to strike because she would get a strange taste in her mouth and would start to see little dots or zigzag lines—not black lines but jagged areas of light and shadow—and couldn't stand bright lights. She'd close the curtains in the middle of the day and when that wasn't dark enough would retreat into her bedroom and draw the curtains.

Zoe suffered from classic migraine with aura. Fortunately, only a small minority of migraine sufferers—perhaps 10 to 20 percent of the total—experience the temporary sensory distortions we call "aura." But Zoe Rosencrantz had all the typical warning symptoms, including a distinct aura about a half-hour before her head pain began. There was never any doubt about her problem.

AURA

For women like Zoe who suffer from migraine with aura, the visual warning symptoms include seeing blind spots or bright lights, zigzag lines, or distorted images about thirty minutes before the headache starts. Aura may be manifested in various ways. Some women may suffer either a partial or near-total loss of vision. That's why you'll sometimes see migraine victims take off their eyeglasses and polish them in the minutes before a headache comes on.

And auras can get far worse than that. Some people see stars flashing as brightly as the sun, while others have dark and bizarre hallucinations. People who have seen halos over human figures believed that these were visions of divine origin. Some claim that Lewis Carroll's bizarre creations in *Alice through the Looking Glass* were inspired by a pre-migraine headache aura.

I once had a patient whose sense of smell was profoundly affected during her aura phase. Before she felt any migraine pain, she smelled a terrible and most repulsive odor in her own body. The odor wasn't real. It was due to a distortion of her sense of smell caused by migraine. But of course she didn't know that. She genuinely thought her body smelled bad. And since she didn't know when the migraine and the odor might strike, she withdrew more and more from public and personal contact for fear of embarrassing her friends and herself. She became a recluse because of this distortion. It was not until she came to us for the pain and we explained that the smell was not real—it was as imagined as a visual hallucination—that she began to emerge from her self-imposed isolation.

FAMILY HISTORY AND THE HEREDITARY FACTOR

Zoe Rosencrantz had another classic indicator of migraine, a family history crowded with loved ones who shared her disorder. Her mother and her cousins all had migraines and so did her sister.

If you have any question in your mind about whether you suffer from migraine, ask about other female members in your family: Did your grandmother or aunt suffer from unexplained illness each month? A family history of migraine is believed to be highly significant in reaching a diagnosis. In 1954 Dr. Harold Wolff and two of his colleagues published a study of 119 individuals with chronic headache. They found three correlations about migraine in families: (1) 69.2 percent of those persons in the study whose parents both had migraine also had migraine; (2) 44.2 percent of those who had one parent with migraine also suffered the headaches; and (3) 28.6 percent of those whose parents didn't have migraine but who had some other relative with migraine, such as an aunt or a cousin, were also plagued by migraines.

One strong school of thought asserts that migraine might

well be the result of a hereditary chemical imbalance that creates a susceptibility to headache triggers that don't bother people without the imbalance. The hormonal changes that occur just before and during menstruation are one such trigger.

But the main chemical many researchers tend to identify as the primary migraine trigger is serotonin. The way in which serotonin is metabolized by the body—that is, how the body handles the substance—seems to be the key. It is believed that migraine is an inherited disorder that somehow affects the way serotonin is metabolized in the body.

THE GENETIC FACTOR

It is also thought that migraine is a genetic disorder which is transmitted through a gene. This premise asserts that a gene passed down through family lines causes migraine, or at least an inclination to migraine. Researchers think that people with the "migraine gene" tend to get headaches when they encounter any one of the migraine triggers, including hormonal changes caused by menstruation, menopause, the Pill, pregnancy, or even certain foods. Moreover, it is within the nature of the genetic code to flash the migraine signal at a certain time. Some people may get the migraine signal in infancy, others in puberty; still others might not get it until their early thirties. Lending credence to this line of thought is the fact that recent studies have identified a possible migraine gene.

MIGRAINE PERSONALITY

Zoe Rosencrantz also had what I've already described as a migraine, or Type A, personality. Generally, a migraine sufferer's personality is described as being perfectionist, orderly, ambitious, cautious, and emotionally repressed; that is, they suppress their feelings of anger or hostility or inadequacy, which other people express readily through emotional explosions. By and large, they are also very bright and alert; they talk very quickly and to the point, and they tend to overload or to expect too much of themselves. What's the connection between personality and migraine? No one knows. We know only that many doctors have reported them in the medical literature, and Zoe's personality seems to fit the migraine pattern.

Now this is not to say that every one of the millions of people who have migraine is exactly like this. Nor is it to say the opposite: that everybody who is like this has migraine. We all know exceptions. My point is that you can look for a migraine personality in people who have a pain in their heads, but the personality is only a clue not a final index of what the pain is all about.

We also know that certain kinds of stress, such as great fear or suddenly inspired excitement, cause an increase in adrenaline in the body that may bring about migraine attacks. But "slower burning" stress like that generated by adjusting to a new job, living in a new city, or even fatigue, hunger, eyestrain, or preparing for a big party may do the same.

In Zoe Rosencrantz, the general migraine personality was pronounced, though not in every final detail. As is typically the case, she would never admit that she wasn't capable of doing whatever she wanted to do. It was simply part of her makeup. She felt that there was no amount of work she couldn't handle and that she could overcome anything that was put in her path. This is one reason why migraine headaches are so frustrating for women like Zoe and why

Biochemistry of Migraine

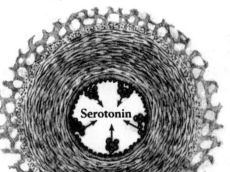

Phase 1. Aura phase

- Platelets release serotonin.
- Blood vessel constriction begins.

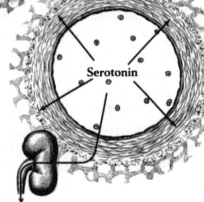

Phase 2. Headache phase

- Serotonin levels begin to decrease.
- Blood vessel dilation begins.
- Blood vessel walls become inflamed.

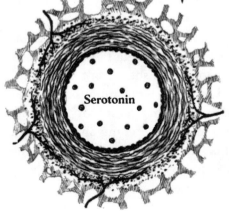

Phase 3. Postheadache phase

- Serotonin levels are normal.
- Blood vessel size returns to normal.
- Blood vessel walls are still inflamed.
- Nerve endings to blood vessel walls are sensitized, resulting in tenderness to touch.

they often hate to admit to anyone that they even have them. For such women, headaches are seen as a sign of weakness they are actually embarrassed about.

There is a theory among some headache experts that a migraine headache indicates that a person is being overloaded, that it's your body's way of telling you to slow down, just as a cold in the nose keeps you huddled inside a warm house instead of hiking through the snow in below-freezing weather.

When headaches like Zoe's continue for fifteen years or more, they have considerable impact on the attitudes of those afflicted with them. Pain literally dominates their lives. They can get nobody else to understand quite how bad it is, while they surrender time and time again to the tyranny of pain. Such women don't live, they just try to exist—from day to day, week to week—wondering when their next headache will strike. They can plan nothing, count on nothing.

As Old as History

Zoe's problem, migraine, was endured for thousands of years before it was labeled. Many famous people have been afflicted by migraine. Frédéric Chopin, Charles Darwin, Leo Tolstoy, Alfred Nobel, Karl Marx, Edgar Allan Poe, Pyotr Ilich Tchaikovsky, and Virginia Woolf are just a few of these. It is said that Queen Mary I—"Bloody Mary"—went to her coronation with a migraine.

The only way we can explain migraine in so many famous and accomplished people is by referring back to some of the elements in the Type A migraine personality: these people are very bright and alert. They are the "doers." They are utterly determined that they are going to achieve a particular goal at a particular time, and nothing, not even a severe and recurring headache, is going to stop them.

Vascular Theory of Migraine

A. Cerebral arteries in normal state. Notice that all the large arteries are surrounded by nerves. When these arteries swell, the nerves send pain stimuli to the brain.

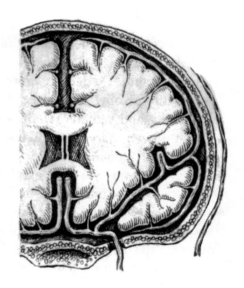

— parenchymal arteries

— pial artery

— scalp artery

— large basal arteries

— extracranial arteries

B. Those cerebral arteries that are surrounded by nerves spasm, resulting in reduced cerebral blood flow. This reduction in blood flow reduces the delivery of oxygen to the area and causes the visual aura sensation associated with migraine.

Vascular Theory of Migraine (continued)

C. In response to reduced blood flow to the brain, the tiny blood vessels without nerves (parenchymal vessels) dilate to try to meet the demands of the brain.

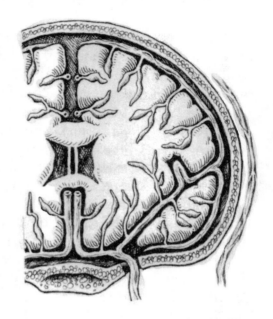

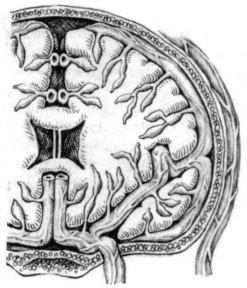

D. Dropping serotonin levels result in dilation of all the arteries. The result is the headache phase of migraine.

THE MYSTERIOUS MECHANISM OF MIGRAINE

The chemical chain reactions that cause migraine headaches appear to be far more complex then those that cause tension headaches. A migraine begins when the blood vessels deep inside the brain constrict. Why do they constrict? Because a hormone called serotonin is excreted by blood platelets.

Platelets are blood components smaller than red blood cells that are part of the body's protective clotting system. If platelets don't stick to each other and the blood vessel walls after an injury, bleeding is dangerously prolonged. But if they clump too quickly, clots may form too readily within the blood vessels. When these clots break loose, heart attack and stroke can result.

In a normally functioning system, the platelets release the hormone serotonin when they begin to clump. As described earlier the presence of serotonin sets off the pro- duction of two other chemicals: thromboxane and prosta- cyclin. Thromboxane goes to work first, helping serotonin to narrow the brain's blood vessels abruptly. The hormonal combination of serotonin and thromboxane dramatically decreases blood flow in the brain and causes the aura stage of migraine.

In the second stage of a migraine attack, serum serotonin levels drop drastically, and the blood vessels of the skull dilate quickly, causing the intense, pounding pain of a migraine headache. The pain is throbbing because the blood pulses through the swollen arteries in time with the pulsing of blood from the heart. Prostacyclin contributes to this process by forcing the blood vessels to dilate still further.

Finally, in the third phase of a migraine (the post- headache phase), the throbbing headache gradually subsides and is replaced by a constant unwavering pain. The blood vessels tend to become thicker and more rigid. As the headache goes on, thromboxane and prostacyclin convert to other hormones, prostaglandins. These cause the artery walls to become inflamed and thicken, often leading to visible swelling of blood vessels on the scalp, temples, or back of the neck. Although the migraine headache is over, the pain isn't. The prostaglandins have also caused the nerve endings in the head and scalp area to become sensitized, often so badly that just combing the hair is painful.

There's an important distinction here between blood vessel dilation and blood vessel inflammation. If you sit in a very hot bath, for example, the blood vessels in your head will dilate, but you won't suffer a pain such as migraine. Similarly, if you exercise long and hard, your blood vessels will dilate without causing pain.

During a migraine attack, however, the blood vessels not only dilate but also become inflamed. It's a sterile inflammation, which means that the blood vessels become inflamed without the presence of infection. (When the skin surrounding a cut becomes very sore and red, the inflammation is usually due to infection.) We believe it is the combination of inflammation and pressure on distended blood vessel walls that causes the pain of migraine.

Despite the fact that the "serotonin-release" theory of migraine has been popular among researchers for more than thirty years, it's clear that the activity of serotonin cannot be the only mechanism that causes migraines.

One study has shown, for example, that when serotonin was administered intravenously, it produced migraine in only eleven of twenty-five migraine patients. And drugs that oppose the actions of serotonin, known as serotonin antagonists, are effective at preventing migraine attacks in only 50 to 60 percent of patients. The reason may be that serotonin is just one of many neurotransmitter hormones in the body. In fact, new transmitters are being discovered at a great rate, said to be one every six weeks.

SUMMARY SHEET: MIGRAINE

Warning Signs: Women who suffer from migraine with aura often experience visual hallucinations about thirty minutes before their headaches start. These hallucinations range from visual blind spots to flashing lights or zigzag lines. Women may also suffer from neurological symptoms such as tingling or numbness in their arms and legs. In migraine without aura, the patient may experience vague premonitions of a headache, such as sudden fatigue or increased energy and appetite. Some women will note strange smells or odors before headache onset. Women with migraine without aura may also note a vague change of mood and mental acuity which predicts their migraine attacks.

Symptoms: Severe one-sided headache, fluid retention, nausea, vomiting, loss of appetite, photophobia, and fatigue.

Unique Symptoms: Menstrual migraine headaches usually occur only immediately before, during, and the first two days after the end of the menstrual flow. Some patients will complain of headache near the time of ovulation. Migraine is not a daily headache.

Typical Duration and Severity: Migraine typically continues from four to twenty-four hours. The length and intensity of migraine attacks are variable. Some women are incapacitated by severe migraine headache and are forced to lie down in a darkened room for the duration of their migraine attack.

Treatment: The most effective prescription drugs for the treatment of menstrual migraines are the nonsteroidal anti-inflammatory agents (NSAIDs). Other drug therapies used to prevent menstrual migraine will be discussed in Chapter 10. Any of these drugs should be started two to three days before menstruation begins and continued throughout the duration of the flow. Abortive therapy, including sumatriptan, ergotamine, or isometheptene, is often helpful after the flow.

Effective Self-Treatments: Biofeedback and relaxation techniques may be helpful in decreasing the severity and duration of migraine attacks. For those with menstrual migraine these techniques should be started two to three days before the period begins and then continued through the duration of the flow. In patients with migraine with aura the techniques should be employed at the first sign or warning of an impending headache. Patients should also identify and avoid headache triggers. All of these will be discussed in later chapters.

When to See Your Doctor: A woman with migraine should consult her physician if the severity of the headache hampers her everyday activities.

5

*H*EADACHE AND *P*REGNANCY

Dr. Mira Buganti was on a straight-arrow course for success. The twenty-seven-year-old resident physician was about to complete her residency at Temple University School of Medicine in Philadelphia and enter into a thriving private practice with her physician husband, Bruce.

Before her attack, Mira's only physical problem was an occasional bout of asthma. Then one night she suddenly developed a splitting headache in her right temple. She was at home in bed, but on call to the hospital. Knowing the signs of a stroke, she wasn't worried that was what it was. Her headache hadn't come on that rapidly. It was just a headache . . . a bad one.

Then her vision became blurred. The headache and the blurred vision lasted for an hour. Still, she wasn't worried until her left hand suddenly went to sleep, with a sensation of numbness, prickling, and tingling. The numbness quickly began creeping up her left arm to her shoulder, then up her neck, eventually incapacitating the left half of her tongue and face.

Bruce was worried. He put her into the car and raced for the hospital in the middle of the night, convinced his wife was suffering from some sort of brain hemorrhage. But by the time they got to the emergency department, the numbness had completely disappeared and an excruciating migraine headache had set in, the first one Mira had ever experienced.

A quick but thorough medical history was taken as doctors raced their young colleague through the most complete set of testing available to modern medicine. Mira had no previous history of headache or abnormal neurological signs, even with the sleep deprivation all too familiar to young resident physicians. There was no family history of migraines. The emergency department doctors looked worried. They, too, feared a stroke.

After five hours of extensive testing, all indicators were normal, and Mira's colleagues were puzzled. Then the serum β-HCG results came back and Mira's mystery ailment was finally diagnosed. She had not realized it, but she was pregnant. A diagnosis of migraine with aura was made. Happily, the rest of her pregnancy went quite normally without another similar incident, and she delivered a healthy child.

Mira's case illustrates why women of child-bearing age who suffer a sudden-onset headache before their menstrual cycle normally begins would be well advised to have a pregnancy test before undergoing more expensive and invasive tests or hospitalization.

RELIEF FOR THE MAJORITY

Although Mira Buganti is by no means an isolated case, most women enjoy welcome relief from their severe headaches during pregnancy. Why does pregnancy seem to confer protection against migraines for most women? The answer seems to be that levels of the female hormones estrogen and progesterone remain fairly constant throughout pregnancy. The wild monthly fluctuations of these hormones before, during, and after the menstrual cycle are temporarily halted during pregnancy. This hormonal lull begins eight to ten days after fertilization, and by the end of the third month most women are free of their migraines until after delivery of their baby.

In a study done in 1959, 80 percent of pregnant women who suffered from migraines before pregnancy noticed improvement during their pregnancy. In another, more detailed study done in 1970 in Australia, involving 200 pregnant women, thirty-one had a history of chronic migraine (15.5 percent). Of the thirty-one migraine sufferers, the headaches completely disappeared in seven women for the duration of their pregnancy (22.6 percent). An additional seventeen women showed some improvement in the number or severity of their headaches. In all, twenty-four of the thirty-one migraine sufferers (77.4 percent) got better during their pregnancy.

The remaining seven migraine sufferers (22.6 percent) didn't get any relief. Their headaches either became more frequent or more severe. In addition, seven other women of the 200 pregnant women studied (3.5 percent) actually developed migraines for the first time as a result of their pregnancy. Migraines began in the first trimester in five women, in the second trimester in one, and in the third trimester in another case.

Why doesn't every woman with migraines get relief during pregnancy? Researchers are not absolutely sure but they think it's because of individual differences in the sensitivity of a woman's estrogen receptors. Located in the hypothalamus gland, these receptors determine how a woman will respond to changing hormone levels. For most women, stabilized estrogen levels during pregnancy decrease headaches although there is some fluctuation in the first trimester. But in some women, because of genetic differences in their estrogen receptors, these same changes actually cause headaches.

SAFETY ISSUES

Since 19 percent of women of childbearing age suffer from migraines, that means millions of women worldwide still suffer attacks during pregnancy. Because the vast majority of these attacks strike in the first trimester of pregnancy, millions of women seek medical intervention for their headaches during this period at the very time when the fetus is most susceptible to drug-induced deformities.

Are these drugs safe, and what treatment options are there for the concerned expectant mother? Researchers tackled the safety issue in a major British study. Scientists looked at 450 female migraine sufferers who had become pregnant and 136 male migraine sufferers whose wives had become pregnant. The assumption was that some percentage of migraine sufferers would have sought drug treatment with the drug of choice at the time, ergotamine tartrate or a similar derivative.

Surprisingly, the malformation rate in the migraine patients studied was 18.5 percent lower than in the control group without headaches, and 9.3 percent lower than the British national average.

This finding is controversial, however. Because ergotamine tartrate and similar derivatives are powerful drugs, I do not recommend them for pregnant women or for people with circulatory or cardiac problems.

All drugs must be *avoided* whenever possible during the first three months of pregnancy. After the first trimester, your obstetrician may consider prescribing preventive drugs or analgesics for acute headaches. However, do not take any drugs without first discussing them with your obstetrician.

NONDRUG THERAPIES FOR PREGNANT WOMEN

There are no self-help techniques that are specific to pregnant women. Please check the last chapter, How To Help Yourself, for ideas such as:

- Biofeedback
- Relaxation training
- Anti-migraine diet: eliminating chocolate, aged cheese, red wine, peanuts, salt, fresh-yeast breads, citrus fruits, meats and cheeses cured with nitrites, alcohol, pork, and lima and navy beans
- Cold packs
- Exercise such as running
- Neck-relaxation exercises

POSTNATAL HEADACHES

After labor and delivery it's very common for new mothers to suffer from headaches. These are called postpartum or postnatal headaches. They are usually tension-type headaches with a generalized, constant pain as the chief complaint.

Migraine sufferers may get migraines as well, although the headaches may be milder than a typical full-blown attack. The headaches seem to correlate with the sharp rise in estrogen and progesterone levels that follows labor and delivery.

In a survey of 100 women at the end of their first post-partum week, 33 percent reported having postnatal headaches in the first seven days following delivery. Postnatal headaches were usually present for more than one day, the average lasting two and one-half days. But the onset of post-natal headaches tended to cluster around the fourth to sixth day after delivery.

As you would expect, most headache sufferers either had a previous history of migraines or a family history of migraines. Among women with either a history of migraines previous to pregnancy or a family history of migraines, 62 percent developed a postnatal headache. Among women with neither a personal or family history of migraine, only 14 percent developed a postnatal headache.

Postnatal headache occurred even when the women had not experienced any migraine episodes for several years. It is very likely that the hormonal shifts that cause migraine are more pronounced after childbirth than the normal ebb and flow associated with the menstrual cycle.

POSTPUNCTURE HEADACHE

In recent years the popularity of spinal blocks, or epidural blocks, to reduce the pain of delivery has been growing. But so have headaches that hours or days later frequently follow spinal-puncture procedures. These headaches can be mild to severe and last a few days or occasionally a few weeks; they strike in about one-quarter of the cases.

The pain is a dull, deep ache and may be throbbing. It usually occurs in the temples in the front of the head or at the base of the skull in the back of the head. If at the base of the skull, it is frequently associated with moderate stiffness of the neck. Characteristic of the pain is that it is virtually eliminated when the patient lies down.

Before the procedure, the patient should discuss needle size with the physician. Using the smallest needle possible may avoid complications associated with lumbar puncture, especially in patients with a history of migraine.

Postpuncture headaches are thought to be caused by spinal fluid that leaks through the puncture site. The best treatment is prevention. Patients should remain lying flat for twelve to twenty-four hours after the procedure. Unfortunately, there's not much we can suggest to relieve this type of headache. It seems to resist most medications. However, that doesn't mean you shouldn't try. Everyone is different. Analgesics may work in your case, but be prepared for a possible long bout with headaches. In some cases symptoms have lasted from two to sixteen weeks. If the headache continues, your physician may perform a blood patch to prevent further leakage of spinal fluid.

You can try the self-help tips in the last chapter, but the only thing that works for most people is resting in bed in the horizontal position and the passage of time.

6

$\mathcal{H}$ EADACHE AND $\mathcal{H}$ ORMONE $\mathcal{P}$ ILLS

Kathy Nelson was a fifty-five-year-old accountant who couldn't shake her migraine attacks. For forty years she had suffered without letup.

Like so many others, she had bounced from doctor to doctor over the years. She had been told that once she went through menopause the headaches would stop. That was her last hope. But menopause had come and gone, and much to her distress the migraines had increased in the previous couple of years until now they were attacking at the rate of two or three a week, a very high frequency.

When she finally came to our clinic, I listened to her story intently then began asking questions. It didn't take long to get to the source of her continuing problem. Kathy had begun taking female hormone pills when she passed through menopause, and she was still taking them.

Migraine headaches usually stop after menopause because there is less fluctuation in the secretion of female hormones in the body. In other words, no hormones, no headaches. But there was no reduction in the fluctuations of Kathy's female hormones after menopause because she was taking female hormone pills.

She refused to give up the hormone pills because she feared a loss of femininity and osteoporosis. For years she had heard of the dangers of osteoporosis and the propensity for hip fractures in women who did not remain on hormone supplements. Despite the fact that I suggested that the hormone tablets might be the cause of her problem, she just couldn't or wouldn't stop taking them.

For more than a year we did the best we could to manage her headaches, largely through use of the ergot-based drugs. But then one day she called me in a state of near panic. Yes, she had migraine pain, but it was much more than that. She had developed a paralysis of her right arm and her right leg. She was convinced that she had suffered a stroke and that the headache might have been more than a migraine. She feared she had broken a blood vessel in her brain; in other words, a stroke.

I had her admitted to the hospital immediately. We ran through some neurological examinations and, sure enough, there was evidence of a "neurological deficiency." Her knee and arm reflexes on the right side were affected and there was a positive Babinski response in her right foot (that is, the big toe bent upward when the bare sole of her foot was stroked instead of bending downward, which is the typical response). In other words, her nervous system wasn't responding typically.

In previous years I would have ordered an angiogram on Kathy. Angiography is an invasive test to have a look inside the body. Unfortunately it can pose a serious threat to the patient. However, the introduction of MRI (magnetic resonance imaging) or MRA (magnetic resonance angiography)

6

has helped us considerably. MRA is a new technique that helps physicians see the blood vessels almost as efficiently as angiography, without the risk of reactions to infused dye. Now we can look inside through the use of very strong magnetic fields without ever having to puncture the skin. Kathy's MRA was negative.

I believed that she had not, in fact, suffered a stroke but a severe episode of complicated, or *hemiplegic*, migraine. However, it is very difficult to distinguish a stroke from complicated migraine, especially in older patients.

Soon we were sure that my diagnosis was correct. We treated Kathy, not for stroke but for complicated migraine. She recovered from her paralysis quickly. The migraine, being deeply involved with the blood vessels around the brain, had merely caused a complication that mimicked the appearance of a stroke. The incident had given her a good scare, though, enough so that I was able to get her off the hormone pills. Within a matter of weeks, her severe headaches dissipated, and now she suffers from only an occasional, very mild migraine.

Kathy Nelson suffered from hemiplegic, or complicated, migraines, which are said to occur when a migraine attack seems to cause neurological changes. The victim notices a numbness in one of her limbs or a partial blindness. In more serious cases there will be a partial paralysis of anything from a muscle in an eyelid to an entire side of the body.

It is often thought to be a stroke, but it is rarely as serious or permanent as that. It is more often a migraine complication masquerading as a stroke. It seems to come on as a result of prolonged change in the concentration of the female hormones of the body, particularly a change that is artificially induced, as in the use of the Pill or female hormones consumed during and after menopause.

ESTROGEN REPLACEMENT THERAPY IN MENOPAUSE

Like Kathy, more and more women are taking female hormone pills to treat or prevent a wide variety of symptoms associated with menopause. These may include irregular or prolonged periods, osteoporosis, hot flashes, excessive sweating, vaginal dryness, and depression. Some women also take hormones to reduce the risk of cardiovascular disease linked to menopause.

Unfortunately, menopause, or the complete ending of ovulation and menstruation, doesn't just happen overnight. A woman's body often goes through changes for months or even years before and after this natural event. A woman's last period usually occurs between the ages of forty and fifty, but can happen as early as thirty-five or as late as sixty. In the years leading up to menopause, her menstrual cycle is disrupted and her periods may become irregular as the ovaries stop producing the female hormones estrogen and progesterone.

About 25 percent of women do not notice any changes at menopause except the cessation of their periods. Another 50 percent undergo slight physical and/or mental changes. The remaining 25 percent experience the discomfort of additional symptoms that include palpitations (irregular heartbeat), joint pains, flushing of the upper torso, and headaches. Other nonphysical symptoms often associated with menopause include depression, anxiety, irritability, decreased ability to concentrate, lack of confidence, and sleeping problems. In light of the fact that such symptoms may last from a few weeks to more than five years, it is easy to see why some women turn to hormone-replacement therapy for relief.

The hormones may be a combination of estrogen and progesterone, or estrogen alone, in the form of tablets, vaginal cream, or a skin patch. Because of so many proven and possible benefits, women tend to overlook the side effects of hormone-replacement therapy. And that can mean terrible headache pain for women, like Kathy Nelson, who are susceptible to migraines.

Migraine during menopause is a complex problem. It used to be thought that migraine disappears with the arrival of menopause but we now know that such is not always the case. Usually migraine prevalence does tend to decrease as women get older. But it can also regress or spontaneously worsen at menopause. This is because in some women any change in amount of estrogen, such as the sudden and significant drop that occurs in menopause, can lead to migraine. In these cases, a small dose of daily estrogen can be helpful.

Women who choose hormone-replacement therapy during menopause should be aware that the hormones may worsen their headaches right away, or prolonged usage may cause them to worsen over time. Research has shown that if hormone therapy does make your headache problem worse, discontinuing the hormones may not bring immediate relief; there may be a delay of several months.

In one interesting case involving hormone-replacement therapy, a forty-eight-year-old woman began suffering terrible migraines one hour after rigorous exercise routines. She had attended aerobics classes three times a week for six years. For the past year, however, she had been struck with severe headaches following every exercise session.

At first the throbbing pain of the post-exercise headaches and the accompanying nausea lasted only a few hours and then subsided with bed rest. But a whopping nine-hour migraine attack, complete with dizziness, finally sent her to her local doctor and a neurologist. After several fruitless neurological tests, she realized that her headaches had begun at the same time that she had switched from oral estrogen replacement pills to the estrogen patch she wore constantly on her buttocks.

The mystery of the post-exercise headaches was solved. When the woman attended her aerobics classes it boosted her blood circulation and increased her absorption of estrogen from the patch on her buttocks. The additional estrogen then triggered a severe headache. When the woman later took off her estrogen patch during her aerobics classes, she had no further headaches.

HORMONE THERAPY AND AURAS

One recent study in Switzerland at the University Eye Clinic at Basel observed that a group of menopausal women who had previously suffered from migraine got more severe headaches within two weeks to three years after starting to wear an estrogen patch. Another group of women who had never gotten migraines began experiencing migraine auras, characterized by blurred vision and other visual disturbances with and without headache, soon after they started using the estrogen patch. The study concluded that estrogen replacement therapy not only triggered more headaches, but also prompted a marked increase of visual auras among migraine-prone women.

For women determined to take female hormones during or after menopause, there are several strategies they can try in an attempt to circumvent hormone-related headaches. First, they should have their doctor determine the lowest dose of estrogen that is effective in controlling their menopausal symptoms. Second, they should take their supplemental hormones continuously, instead of using an interrupted schedule in which estrogens are taken for twenty-five days each month. One study reports a 58 percent improvement in headache control when women switched to a reduced, continuous dose of estrogen.

ORAL CONTRACEPTIVES

The Pill tends to increase the frequency, duration, severity, and complications of migraine by exacerbating the fluctuations of female hormones in the body. Women who are sensitive to such hormonal changes experience vascular changes that make them more vulnerable to migraines. This vulnerability is most noticeable in women who have already shown a tendency to get migraines in the first place.

In fact, migraine headaches are the most common side effect reported by those taking the Pill. Overall, the headache-producing effects of the Pill cause women to stop taking it more often than most doctors realize. In one study, more than one-quarter of the women taking the Pill stopped because the frequency and intensity of their migraines had become intolerable.

In 1977 even more interesting research was published. French researchers studied more than 1,000 women who had been using the Pill for more than a year. They concluded that there was no doubt that the use of the Pill aggravates headaches. But they also found something else: that the longer women took the Pill, the fewer headaches they had. In other words, the body may be able to adjust to this artificial input of female hormones—at least as far as headache production goes.

If you have headaches but insist on continuing oral contraceptives, I recommend one of the NSAIDs, starting on the twentieth day of the cycle. You usually remain off the Pill from the twenty-first to the twenty-eight day. Stay on the NSAIDs through the second day of the next cycle.

The Pill is even likely to induce nonvascular headaches. In migraine-free women, the headache pain is not over-whelming; it is usually mild enough that the individual can tolerate it with over-the-counter analgesics.

For the migraine victim it's a different story. Her headaches are likely to increase in severity and frequency when she is on the Pill. If she is getting one or two attacks a month, she may suddenly find herself getting four or six or eight attacks a month after going on the Pill. Or if her migraine headache lasted for twenty-four hours before, she may find it lasting two or three days after she goes on the Pill. Among some migraine-suffering women, the headaches become so frequent and long-lasting that there seem to be fewer and fewer moments during the month when they aren't suffering from migraine.

Moreover, birth control pills can touch off attacks of migraine in women who are susceptible to the problem but who have never before, or very rarely, suffered from it. Unfortunately it doesn't take an enormous concentration of female hormones to touch off migraine in those prone to it.

I had one patient in her thirties who recently had been stricken with severe migraine headaches. Melinda's attacks came every day—very unusual for migraines—and were quickly growing in intensity. Although I couldn't determine the cause for the attacks, I prescribed medications and put her on a special diet.

Melinda had never been on the Pill. But nothing we rec-ommended or prescribed seemed to work. Her headaches continued to grow more ferocious.

It was a baffling case. I spent long hours checking and

rechecking every conclusion I had made. Then one day I noticed that Melinda worked for a drug company.

"They're famous for their birth control pills," I commented casually.

"Yes," she said. "I know. I work in the section where the pills are made."

I couldn't believe it. That was it!

She was breathing in tiny particles of the birth control pills suspended in the air. And as we know, the estrogen in the Pill is a cause for migraine headaches. I wrote to the company and explained the problem. She was reassigned to another division, and her headaches ceased altogether.

Beyond all this, the impact of the elements in the Pill exposes migraine patients to complications that might escalate into problems of dramatic proportions. We have noticed, for example, the reports of several investigators pointing out the increased number of strokes among rather young women who have migraine. What they had most in common, besides their migraine, was taking birth control pills. Numerically the group of apparent stroke victims was not large, but the circumstances and coincidence were striking. Although the incidence is admittedly low, the impact of pill-related stroke is dramatic on those who represent the statistic.

7

*T*ENSION-TYPE *H*EADACHES

Sister Bridget Ward was one of my favorite patients. She always had a ready smile and a firm handshake. At her office visits the first few minutes were spent with Sister Bridget asking how I was feeling and if I was taking care of myself. When Sister Bridget first came to see me, she was a member of a large religious order and taught eighth grade in a Chicago parochial school. She herself looked about fourteen, although she was thirty-two at the time of her first visit. I could imagine her playing basketball with her students or dancing at a prom. Sister Bridget was full of life except for the two or three days each month when she had her migraine attacks.

Sister Bridget's headache history was fairly typical. Her migraine attacks started at age fourteen and were usually linked to her period. She did not experience an aura prior to an attack, but she did complain of severe nausea and vomiting associated with the headache. Her mother, maternal grandmother, and all three of her sisters had similar histories of migraine attacks. If she indulged in a pizza after a volleyball game or enjoyed a bit of chocolate candy, she could expect a migraine attack. Sister Bridget took an NSAID at the start of menses, and she used an ergot suppository when she felt a headache starting.

Her visits were scheduled on a semimonthly basis for about two years, until Sister Bridget came in with a variety of additional complaints. She was experiencing a migraine attack every week, and she felt twinges of a headache on a daily basis. Furthermore, she was waking daily at 4 A.M., and couldn't go back to sleep. I knew that something was wrong and questioned her about her new teaching position at a coed high school in suburban Detroit. The transfer was not a joyous one. Sister Bridget's family lived on the north side of Chicago, and her parents were both in poor health. She had enjoyed the camaraderie at her old school and parish, and she now faced living in a large community of sisters in an area in which she felt totally a stranger.

The biggest problem was a mother superior who ran the convent like a marine barracks. Sister Bridget was facing a major dilemma in her life, a life that she had chosen for herself at age eighteen. Many of the issues she was encountering were similar to those of someone going through a divorce. I could provide Sister Bridget with medications, but she had to confront her problems personally. To treat her coexisting migraine and tension-type headaches, I started her on medications to help both the pain and the sleep disturbance. I also asked Sister Bridget to return to the Clinic in six weeks.

On her next visit, she noted a vast improvement in her headache and sleeping problems. Also, she had asked for a leave of absence to care for her mother, who was recovering from a stroke. The change of scenery was doing wonders for

Sister Bridget's frame of mind. When her father died a few months later, Sister Bridget decided to ask for a release from her religious vows. She would live at her mother's home and look for a job at one of the local parochial schools. During the next four years, Sister Bridget—now simply Ms. Bridget Ward—would stop all of her medications except for the NSAIDs at menses. She was very content with her life and the status of her headaches.

Such headaches are classified as chronic tension headaches. Stress-caused tension headaches often strike

Muscles of the Head

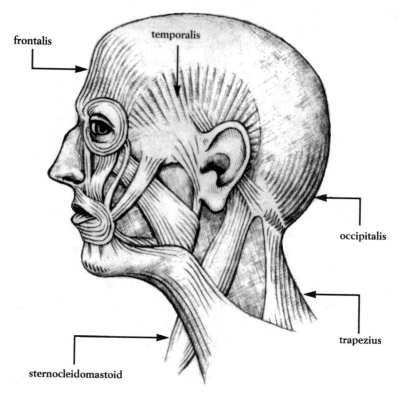

frontalis

temporalis

occipitalis

trapezius

sternocleidomastoid

when you can't vent your anxiety or anger. But they can also hit you when you are just anticipating an unpleasant event. Strangely enough these headaches may actually be absent during the time of high anxiety or stress only to strike later when you are ready to relax. Most of the time, however, they are brought on by stressful situations.

In fact, the common tension headache is really a remnant of the body's wondrous fight-or-flight mechanism. When you feel threatened, your muscles tighten, digestion is slowed, and the heart speeds up. This is your body's way of sharpening your senses and maximizing the amount of energy the body can put to immediate use. When the action is over, the tension is released and everything returns to normal. Right? It's not so simple in our modern world.

Though physical dangers rarely threaten our lives these days, the stress generated by our frenetic lifestyles can cause the same reactions. In today's world, the fight-or-flight reaction to stress is normally counterproductive, because stressful situations are frequently lifestyle related and are not easily resolved. Tense muscles remain tense, and the result can be tension-type headaches, which were previously called muscle-contraction headaches.

What causes tension-type headaches? When you are exposed to stress, the muscles in your jaw, face, scalp, and neck continuously contract and cramp, creating a dull, diffuse, pressure-like pain over the top of the head, temples, or back of the neck. The pain is typically described as a dull, nagging, non-throbbing pressure that feels like a tight band around the head. Contraction and tenderness of the muscles can often be felt just by touching them. Tension headaches lack the sharp, intense, throbbing quality of migraine pain, which usually strikes only one side of the head. In contrast, tension-type headaches are characterized by pain in both

Prostaglandin Production

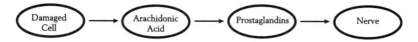

Without aspirin (above), a damaged cell produces arachidonic acid. When arachidonic acid combines with oxygen in the blood, it results in the production of prostaglandins. (Below) Aspirin breaks the chain of chemical reactions that produce pain-enhancing prostaglandins.

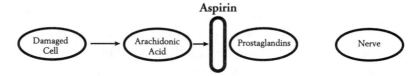

sides of the head as the major arteries in the scalp also clamp down and constrict.

When the muscles of your scalp and neck tighten in response to physical or emotional stress, the flow of blood and oxygen to those muscles becomes restricted. When muscles are tensed over long periods of time, it causes oxygen starvation, or ischemia of the muscles. Because of the lack of oxygen, muscle cells secrete powerful hormone-like substances that further enhance the sensation of pain. It's our body's way of telling us to do something to eliminate the muscle tension, or more pain will follow.

One of those chemicals is arachidonic acid. When activated by an enzyme, it combines with oxygen in the blood to produce prostaglandins. These prostaglandins are hormone-like substances that sensitize the nerve endings to pain. This allows even small concentrations of pain-inducing substances such as serotonin, bradykinin, and others, to start the pain signal on its way.

Aspirin interrupts the conversion of arachidonic acid into nerve-sensitizing prostaglandins and is therefore effective in controlling tension-type headache pain. Believe it or not, it took scientists until 1971 to figure that out—some seventy years after aspirin came into use.

As in other types of headaches, it is your hormones that control the biochemical changes that culminate in tension headache. The adrenal hormones are usually a major culprit. That's because the adrenal glands spring into action, pumping out hormones that stimulate the body's fight-or-flight response whenever we experience stress. Your heart beats faster, your blood pressure rises, and the blood flowing through your small blood vessels slows as they constrict to prevent bleeding from a potential injury. But these responses represent just a fraction of the myriad hormonal changes that occur when a person is subjected to emotional or physical stress.

When a stress-producing situation persists over an extended period of time, the adrenal glands stay abnormally active, continuously "pumping you up" with the very hormones that keep you in a stressed-out state. If you find yourself in a job you hate, teamed-up with difficult coworkers, being ordered around by a boss you resent, or locked into a marriage fraught with conflict, you will probably become all too familiar with tension headaches.

The connection between stress and ill health is well established. Studies show that people who experience a great amount of stress also tend to experience a great amount of illness. In the 1960s psychiatrists Thomas H. Holmes, M.D., and Richard H. Rahe, M.D., at the University of Washington in Seattle created a now-famous checklist of stressful events, which incorporated the very valid concept that any major change in your life, good *or* bad, stresses the body. They ranked major life events for their stress contents. For example, the most negative life events, such as the death of a spouse, led the way as the most stressful, with a rating of 100. Perhaps the most interesting aspect of their work, however, was that even events normally considered positive, like marriage, could also be considered very stressful. Holmes and Rahe found that the higher your total stress score throughout the year, the more likely you were to become seriously ill in the immediate future.

Until recently, people were told to *avoid* stressful events in order to stay physically and mentally healthy. But that's nearly impossible to do in today's world. Everyone has to deal with stress—even "positive stress"—every single day. That means in order to avoid or prevent tension headaches, you have to learn how to cope with stress.

The stress that precipitates these headaches can be either of a short- or long-term nature. Short-term mental or physical stress, like studying for an exam, meeting a deadline, getting a verbal reprimand from your boss, or just missing lunch, can precipitate periodic tension headaches. But as you might guess, long-term emotional stress—a depression or anxiety—that isn't resolved can result in chronic tension headaches that may strike every single day for years.

Almost everyone has experienced the occasional tension headache at one time or another. Such headaches are easily controlled with over-the-counter analgesics and do not continue for days or weeks. Many times these headaches are in response to a short-term stressful situation, fatigue, or a missed meal. Episodic tension-type headaches are usually controllable and not dangerous. Common drugs like aspirin can interrupt the chemical reactions that cause the pain. Since the episodic form is easily controlled, physicians are not usually consulted for these headaches. Those suffering from chronic tension-type headaches should consider, in addition to drugs, an alternative therapy such as biofeedback.

Chronic tension-type headaches usually occur on a daily or almost-daily basis. Although such chronic tension headaches lack the severity of migraines, the frequency and duration of these headaches put patients at risk of developing habituation problems with analgesics. To avoid this, you need to go one level deeper than merely treating symptoms. You need to eliminate the cause of the muscle tension in the first place.

For example, women with chronic tension-type headaches will often complain of trouble sleeping. The headaches themselves are not usually bad enough to wake a person, but the accompanying depression or anxiety does cause sleeping problems. If the headaches are due to anxiety, a woman may notice that she has difficulty falling asleep. If the headaches are related to depression, however, she may complain of frequent or early awakening. It is essential to determine the emotional root of these headaches before selecting therapy.

DEPRESSION

As in Bridget Ward's case there is usually an emotional trigger behind chronic tension-type headaches. Fortunately, Bridget was able to find some relief.

Emotional factors that can cause chronic tension-type headaches include depression, chronic anxiety, stress, suppressed anger, worry, frustration, and fear. When depression is a factor, it is often of such depth that the sufferer does not even know that she is depressed. She thinks that this is the way life is to be lived and therefore associates the accompanying headaches with some past illness or injury. Such depression is not just a "feeling blue" sensation but a serious and lengthy depression that can last for years.

Research of brain chemistry has indicated that when someone is depressed, hormones that act as neurotransmitters, including serotonin, norepinephrine, and others, become depleted. In migraine, a sudden rise in serotonin can trigger the headache. In tension-type headaches, too little of these vital neurotransmitters can cause depression and therefore headaches. These chemicals are necessary for the nervous system to send the nerve impulses from one cell to the next. When adequate concentrations of these chemicals are not present, the nervous system cannot perform its functions. Furthermore, depending on which areas of the brain are affected, a lack of serotonin and the other neurotransmitting hormones can cause disturbances of sleep, appetite, mood, and pain regulation. This is thought to be the reason patients with depression have chronic headache.

Headaches associated with depression establish a regular pattern, occurring primarily in the early morning and early evening. Chronic, tension-type headaches most often occur in the hours from 4:00 A.M. to 8:00 A.M. and from 4:00 P.M. to 8:00 P.M. As I mentioned before, a woman suffering from depression tends to awaken early in the morning or at frequent intervals during the night, preoccupied with the conflict she is experiencing.

Obviously, the most common causes of depression are related to job conflicts and family relationships. The depression itself can be disabling although it often varies in intensity. Depression can cause a slowing down of all of one's functions, or it can take the form of abnormal agitation. Women suffering from depression have many accompanying emotional and physical complaints. They often have difficulty concentrating or remembering things, lose interest easily, and cannot make decisions. Fatigue, weakness, irritability, and suicidal feelings are typically present, as well as a decrease in sexual activity.

Other symptoms of depression include stomach problems, constipation, loss of weight, or lack of appetite. Women struggling with depression complain of feeling sad and may be introverted. A posttraumatic headache is usually put into this category because patients often suffer depression after a head injury, and it is the depression that most often causes posttraumatic headache.

OTHER CAUSES

Chronic tension-type headaches may also be a sign of anxiety. Those headaches caused by anxiety tend to strike unpredictably, at almost any time, unlike depression headaches, which establish a regular pattern, although there is an increase in the severity of anxiety headaches in the mornings, and an increase in the number of such headaches on weekends and holidays. But regardless of whether they are caused by depression or anxiety, both of these chronic tension-type headaches share certain traits. Simple analgesics do not curb their pain.

Occasional or episodic tension-type headaches can also be caused by poor posture, close work under poor lighting conditions, or cramps from assuming an unnatural head position or rigid neck position for long periods of time. Arthritis, primarily cervical arthritis, can also provoke tension-type headaches, as well as pain from other places such as the neck, eyes, and teeth. Disturbances in the neck muscles, bones, or discs can precipitate tension-type headaches, as can abnormal conditions in facial organs. Talk to your doctor about your work and home environments to determine if they are affecting your head pain.

TREATMENT

Chronic tension-type headache sufferers whose headaches occur daily or on an almost daily basis should seek medical help. Such headaches warrant medical intervention because their presence may be symptomatic of some other disease, which should be thoroughly checked out.

Certain forms of psychological, physical, pharmacological, or biofeedback therapy may be very helpful in chronic tension headache treatment. Different types of therapy can be combined in order to bring the head pain under control. Occasionally, one type of therapy will have to replace another treatment approach because of the side effects or negative results experienced from the first type. Keep in mind that one kind of therapy may be beneficial for one individual, while a different form will be more successful for another person.

Although the pain of the every-once-in-a-while kind of tension headache responds to simple analgesics like aspirin, the pain of chronic tension headaches does not. This kind of headache problem has numerous causes and provoking factors. In addition to treating the symptom of head pain, it is also necessary to find the root of the problem. That's why a multifaceted approach works best in the treatment of chronic tension-type headaches. Episodic tension headache, occurring infrequently, does not need more than simple analgesics.

Pharmacological Approaches

There are two types of drugs used in the treatment of chronic tension-type headaches: antidepressants or a non-habituating tranquilizer, buspirone (BuSpar), which reduces tension and anxiety. Antidepressants enable headache sufferers to more easily tolerate and function with their pain until their underlying emotional problems can be dealt with. The antidepressants have an inherent pain-relieving capability that is especially helpful for patients with headache and other chronic pain problems.

The goal of treatment is to slowly decrease and phase out medication as a patient learns to cope with his or her individual situation.

PHYSICAL APPROACHES

Avoiding situations or conditions that involve distortion or rigidity of posture can help to alleviate some tension-type headaches. Many sufferers have found careful exercise and massage of tight neck muscles effective. Heat applied to the neck area may also be helpful, as heat is a muscle relaxant.

PSYCHOLOGICAL APPROACHES

Since emotional factors so often play a role in chronic tension-type headaches, sufferers need to assess their marital, social, and work relationships, along with their personality traits and modes of handling stress. It is necessary for a patient to determine which elements in his or her life are provoking the headaches. It must be emphasized that it is important to find any emotional triggers for the headaches in order to seek a long-term solution to the headache problem and not just temporary treatment of the symptoms. But isolating stress factors can be difficult, since a patient may not even be aware of them.

It may take time to discover the cause of a depression or anxiety headache. Some physicians will treat the headache and others will treat the depression, but one must realize that the headache is part of the depression, and it should be treated as such. For many sufferers, trying to relieve the depression will also alleviate the painful headache symptom. Because a chronic tension-type headache sufferer is likely to be in pain nearly every day, with an accompanying effect on the emotions, a circular phenomenon is often set in motion. Pain provokes emotional upset which triggers more pain, which prompts more emotional upset. Treatment will necessitate interrupting this cycle. Both relaxation training and biofeedback have been shown to be effective.

TREATING DEPRESSION HEADACHES

An antidepressant is the drug of choice for a chronic tension-type headache due to depression. Among women with chronic tension-type headaches due to depression, there is a significant decrease in catecholamines, the group of hormones that includes norepinephrine and dopamine. Researchers have found that treatment that increases or preserves the level of catecholamines in the brain can help to control this type of headache.

Antidepressants seem to work by helping to preserve catecholamines in the brain. They include the following medications: amitriptyline (Elavil, Endep), protriptyline (Vivactil), nortriptyline (Aventyl), imipramine (Tofranil), desipramine (Norpramin), doxepin (Sinequan), venlafaxine (Effexor), fluoxetine (Prozac), maprotiline (Ludiomil), bupropion (Wellbutrin), paroxetine (Paxil), and sertraline (Zoloft).

If your doctor prescribes antidepressants, you'll have to be patient since they may take several weeks to show their effectiveness. Some of the possible side effects include drowsiness, dryness of the mouth, tingling fingers, and blurred vision. Changes in pulse, heart rhythm, blood pressure, and behavior may also occur.

The Monoamine Oxidase Inhibitors (MAOIs) are a form of antidepressants that slow down the metabolism of catecholamines, thus preserving them. It is suspected that both MAOIs and other antidepressants may not only relieve the depression but may also raise the pain threshold. As with migraine headache sufferers on these drugs, chronic tension-type headache patients taking MAOIs must be very careful to avoid foods containing tyramine and all alcoholic beverages to prevent a blood-pressure crisis.

TREATING ANXIETY HEADACHES

The anxiety headache should be treated with a non-habituating tranquilizing drug, buspirone, and limited use of mild pain relievers. These agents will not abort an already existing headache, although they may help the sufferer relax. Tranquilizers may aid in counteracting the tension that provokes many tension-type headaches. They appear to work by raising the sufferer's pain threshold and lessening her reactivity to stress.

Medications known as muscle relaxants are also used in the treatment of tension-type headaches. They are often used in combination with other medications. Muscle relaxants may relieve the muscle spasms that result from excessive contraction of the scalp, face, and neck muscles, thus helping to control the ensuing tension-type headache.

COEXISTING MIGRAINE AND TENSION-TYPE HEADACHES

The majority of women seen at a specialized headache clinic such as the Diamond Headache Clinic are suffering from a combination of migraine and tension-type headaches. This condition is referred to as mixed headache syndrome. Such women usually report an earlier history of recurrent migraine headaches, which tend to strike more and more frequently as time goes on. Once this happens, most of these women note the development of a daily or almost daily headache of milder severity. Due to the frequency of their headaches, these women are particularly prone to dependency problems with analgesics. Because these women have a difficult, dual problem, the routine care for their headaches is usually not sufficient. Their next step would be to seek sophisticated treatment from a neurologist or a headache clinic.

SUMMARY SHEET: TENSION-TYPE HEADACHES

Types: There are two types of tension-type headaches: episodic or chronic. The episodic form is a recurrent headache, usually triggered by stress, fatigue, or other physical factors (e.g., missed meal, poor posture). However, the patient with chronic tension-type headaches will note that these headaches occur on a daily basis and are continuous throughout the day.

Symptoms: Sufferers of both types of tension-type headache experience pain on both sides of the head. The pain is described as a tight headband or a vise around the head. These headaches may be accompanied by tightness or soreness in the neck and shoulders.

In chronic tension-type headaches, the patient will experience a continuous headache. The patient may appear anxious or depressed and may describe a sleep disturbance. In patients with headaches due to anxiety, they may be experiencing difficulty falling asleep. Frequent and early awakening are often seen in patients with chronic tension-type headaches due to depression. These patients may have a multitude of symptoms, in addition to headaches, including chronic fatigue, loss of sexual drive, decreased concentration, diminished memory, easily frustrated, loss of appetite or weight gain, and depressed mood.

Treatment: Episodic tension-type headaches are easily controlled with over-the-counter analgesics, and the patient will rarely consult a physician. For patients with chronic tension-type headaches, preventive therapy is essential. First, the physician must determine the basis for these headaches— anxiety or depression. If the chronic tension-type headaches are due to anxiety, preventive treatment is limited to a mild tranquilizing agent or psychological treatment. For the acute headaches, the patient should only use mild non-habituating analgesics.

Therapy for headaches due to depression may involve the use of antidepressants. A specific type of antidepressant, the monoamine oxidase inhibitors (MAOIs), may be used in those patients who have not responded to the other forms of antidepressants.

If the emotional and psychological factors are profoundly impacting on the patient's headache and life, psychological testing and counseling should be considered. Marital and/or family therapy may also be considered.

8

SEXUAL HEADACHES

Jane Streeter came into my office complaining of two kinds of headaches. One had started at the age of fifteen. The pain affected one side of her head and struck once or twice a month, lasting one to two days. The headache was severe, and she had a history of seeing jagged lines in one eye before many of the headaches started. She also had intense nausea, vomiting, and some photosensitivity with the headache—a classic case of migraine.

The second type of headache had started about six months before her visit and had its first occurrence during sexual excitement. Since then, she had experienced similar sexual headaches five other times. Her sexual headache did not occur with all episodes of intercourse but seemed to develop slowly during sexual activity, reaching its greatest intensity at the moment of orgasm.

The headache was located occipitally, that is at the base of the skull in the back of the head, in contrast to her migraines. Her sexual headache was also bilateral—the pain was on both sides of the head—and involved her neck. She described the pain as dull and cramping in quality, but on two occasions it had been throbbing and severe although not as excruciating as her migraine attacks.

Unlike her migraines, there was no nausea, vomiting, nor aura connected with this headache. The headache always seemed to be related to a particular degree of sexual excitement and took almost seven hours to subside. During these headaches, she noticed that her heart was beating rapidly and that she had throbbing in the ears and a flushed facial feeling. Worried by the unusual symptoms, Jane had a complete neurological examination, but the findings were normal. Because of the exertional nature of the headache, a CT-scan with infusion was also performed, the results of which came back completely normal.

After taking a complete medical history, I began to hone in on Jane's emotional life. It was apparent that she was under stress, trying to balance the demands of teenage children against those of a mushrooming business. But that wasn't enough. Sure, she was under tension, but she appeared capable of dealing with it. There had to be something else. Finally, I asked a very delicate question—about infidelity. Sure enough, there had been an incident; Jane was deeply guilt ridden over the experience, and the guilt was gradually eating away at her. Once the truth was out, the details tumbled from her as though she were anxious to expel them once and for all.

To counter Jane's anxiety I prescribed biofeedback, and she did very well. She soon mastered relaxation of the head, neck, and facial muscles with instructions to use the technique the next time she made love with her husband. You see, in many cases, inner turmoil is not so easily masked as the patient nears orgasm. This pattern of contraction can clearly be responsible for headaches, especially those located at the base of the skull. In one study, seven of ten patients suffering from sexual headaches who also developed tension headaches in other circumstances reported that the nature of the two types of headaches was similar.

In any case, Jane attacked biofeedback training with her usual drive, mastering it in just a few sessions. During the next sexual encounter with her husband, everything went well, and Jane's headaches soon disappeared.

Sex-based headaches can occur at any stage of the sexual act. They are troubling because they can come on abruptly and with great intensity. The sudden appearance of a headache during sexual intercourse, particularly at the time of orgasm, naturally causes a great deal of anxiety. A woman may fear she is about to die of a brain hemorrhage. Although this can indeed happen, such cases are rare. Actually, sexual headaches are usually benign, especially if you've had them before.

It is the profound hormonal changes that occur during sex that trigger this kind of headache. In response to the adrenal hormone activity associated with sexual arousal, your heart rate speeds up and your blood vessels constrict, resulting in blood pressure that can double, up to as high as 220/120 during orgasm. These same adrenal hormones cause your muscles to constrict. But with the exception of some residual heart rhythm irregularities, everything becomes normal again in less than two minutes after orgasm.

Such rapid physiological changes can certainly cause the exertion headaches that sometimes result from a sudden increase in physical activity. But researchers now suspect that sexual headaches frequently have a psychological component as well. In other words, emotional stress (anxiety, depression, anger, guilt, or sorrow) amplifies the normal effect of the adrenal gland's catecholamine hormones, such as adrenaline and noradrenaline, that are circulating in the blood in response to the physical activity associated with sex.

Of course, the secretion of catecholamine hormones during any intense physical activity, including sexual intercourse, is perfectly normal. The same is true of short-lived stress like driving in rush hour traffic or having a fight with your spouse. But health problems arise when the stress, either physical or emotional, persists over long periods of time, leaving the body in a perpetual state of adrenal arousal.

If a woman with a predisposition to headache engages in sex when she is under stress, she is essentially getting a double dose of adrenal hormones, especially if she has been experiencing that stress for a prolonged time. The excessive output of adrenal hormones intensifies the normal strain that sexual activity places on the circulatory system, and headaches during orgasm can result. But a woman's circulatory system is not the only part of her body that is affected by abnormally high catecholamine levels.

Even stress-free sexual activity involves a great deal of catecholamine-controlled muscle contraction that ultimately culminates in orgasm. The muscles of the neck and jaw become progressively tighter as a woman nears climax. During orgasm itself, she may frown, scowl, or grimace as her facial muscles contract involuntarily in semi-spasm. The jaws frequently clench spastically, as do the muscles of the neck. That's because orgasm is an involuntary reflex during which there is a sudden release of the muscular tension and congested blood vessels produced by sexual stimulation.

This is the reason that unresolved emotional stress, and the adrenal hormone output such prolonged stress generates, predisposes women to tension headaches during sex. If the muscles of a woman's neck, jaw, and face are already tight due to stress-related adrenal hormone arousal, the natural muscle contraction that accompanies sexual excitation may cascade into the muscle cramping that triggers the pain of a tension headache.

Personality type also could hormonally predispose certain women to sexual headaches. Studies have found that people who are hyper-reactors, such as time-driven, overly competitive Type A personalities, secrete large amounts of catecholamines in response to even very minor stresses. This chronic overreaction and consequent surge of stress-related hormones would make women of this type more susceptible to headaches during sex.

Other hormones involved in sexual response are the pituitary hormones prolactin, thyroid-stimulating hormone (TSH), adrenal-cortex-stimulating hormone (ACTH), and vasopressin. Studies show that prolactin levels are elevated during sexual response and during migraine attacks as well. Similarly, higher levels of estrogen are associated with both increased sexual response and headache. This is thought to be one of the reasons that chronic headaches tend to disappear after menopause, when the ovaries diminish production of estrogen and estrogen levels remain low and stabilized.

Prolactin, ACTH, and TSH are referred to as trophic hormones because they stimulate other glands or organs to go into action. During foreplay, or the first stage of sexual arousal, for example, the parasympathetic part of the nervous system promotes the relaxation of blood vessels. The hormone vasopressin causes the muscular walls of blood vessels to relax and expand so that blood can collect and pool in the veins of the clitoris and surrounding areas. This blood becomes trapped like a balloon that has been tied at one end. As part of this process, the pituitary hormone ACTH orders the adrenal glands to produce the hormone cortisol, which speeds up the body's metabolic rate. The pituitary hormone TSH also tells the thyroid to accelerate metabolism.

As the sensation of sexual arousal builds, the sympathetic

nervous system asserts itself. The adrenal glands secrete the catecholamine hormones, adrenaline and noradrenaline, which elevate heart rate and blood pressure still further. These adrenal hormones reverse the dilation of clitoral blood vessels and force the muscular layer of these veins to constrict instead. The blood pressure within the region grows to such an extent that it triggers the involuntary reflex we call orgasm, during which there is a sudden release of muscular tension and congested blood vessels.

Unlike migraines, sexual headaches are normally bilateral, that is, both sides of the head hurt. They fall into three basic classifications: pre-orgasm, mid-orgasm, and postcoital.

Headaches that occur during orgasm are usually caused by high blood pressure or exertion. Such head pain constitutes the most worrisome form of sexual headache because it usually comes on so abruptly and with such intensity. Unlike the pulsating pain of many migraines, these headaches are usually described as "contusive," that is, as though someone hit you on the back of the head with a lead pipe.

Orgasmic headaches usually require careful screening for any one of several serious organic diseases. That's why we checked out Jane so thoroughly. It cannot be stressed enough, however, that if you experience repetitive sexual headaches which occur with orgasm, you *must* see your doctor. Serious diseases must be ruled out first.

Once your doctor has given you a clean bill of health, the nonsteroidal anti-inflammatory agents (NSAIDs) can be successfully used to treat exertional headaches, including orgasmic headaches. These drugs can be used as daily preventive medications or for acute therapy at the onset of a major headache.

DURATION

Headaches that occur during the early stages of foreplay or intercourse are brief, usually lasting for only a few minutes, except when they herald a brain hemorrhage. The duration of orgasmic headaches is variable. In most patients, the extreme pain lasts only ten to fifteen minutes, but in one study, over one-third of patients suffered from pain lasting from one hour to several hours. Postcoital headaches are often lengthy, persisting for several hours or even days.

Sexual headaches are often repetitive. The number of repetitions and their recurrence vary from patient to patient. The most troubling time is the first occurrence. You are worried about an aneurysm, and rightly so. The bottom line is if you have had it before, don't worry.

In one study, over 50 percent of patients had experienced sexual headaches two to three times. About 15 percent of patients got a headache one out of five times they had sex. The remaining 30 percent of patients got the headaches almost every time they had sex.

BRAIN HEMORRHAGE

About 10 percent of sexual headaches have a serious disorder as the cause. Seeing your physician is a must to rule out a catastrophic illness.

The high blood pressures and heart rates associated with sexual activity are sometimes the triggering mechanism for a ruptured blood vessel or aneurysm. Unfortunately there are rarely warning signs of this type of headache. You either have it and are in desperate need of immediate medical attention, or you don't.

MARITAL FIDELITY

One of the most interesting aspects of sexual headaches is that both brain hemorrhages and heart attacks occur much less frequently during sex between couples who have been married for a long time than during sexual activity with new partners. This is because the excitement of illicit sex is often much greater and presents a greater level of stress on the individuals engaging in it. Likewise, the cardiovascular strain caused by intercourse has been found to be modest in middle-aged, long-married couples.

On the other hand, at least one study has shown that married individuals who deny the presence of emotional stress in their lives and refuse to seek psychotherapy have a low response rate to medicine, biofeedback, and dietary changes. That's why it is important for headache sufferers to undergo a marital assessment evaluation. Such evaluations can pinpoint trouble areas in the marriage that need to be addressed during counseling.

The following questions might be asked of each marriage partner, separately, during such an evaluation:

- When did the headaches begin? Did they occur before or after marriage? Have the headaches increased in frequency, duration, intensity, or disability since being married?

- What begins or contributes to the headaches?

- What can you do to help reduce the frequency, duration, intensity, or disability of the headaches?

- How does your spouse react to you when you have a headache? What do you do when your spouse has a headache?

- How do the headaches affect you? How do the headaches affect your spouse? How do the headaches affect your relationship with your spouse?

Depending on the results of the interview, it can be determined whether marital therapy is indicated in conjunction with standard headache therapy. Gauging the headache sufferers' and their spouses' level of marital adjustment and offering marital therapy to those who need it boosts the success rate of headache treatments of all types.

TREATMENT

It cannot be stated too strongly that any type of orgasmic, sexual, or stress headache needs, above all, an examination and a thorough workup to rule out catastrophic causes of headache.

Generally speaking, drug therapy is particularly helpful in patients with orgasmic headache. Where psychological and relationship issues are present, the use of biofeedback and counseling should be instituted.

Frequently the best course of action to prevent sexual headaches is something you can do on your own. Here are eight techniques you can try:

1. If you feel a dull headache coming on during sexual activity, try stopping. Orgasm usually aggravates the headache. Your body may be issuing a warning to try it again at a later time.

2. Take a more passive role during intercourse.

3. Lose weight and exercise more. We suspect that a general state of poor cardiovascular fitness can be a contributing factor.

4. Try increasing the duration of sexual activity, especially prolonging the excitement stage before orgasm. What you are doing is giving your body more time to adjust to sexual activity gradually. It could reduce the huge spikes in blood pressure, heart rate, and possibly hormonal output that may be causing your headache.

5. Limit abrupt body movements or postural changes.

6. Slow down or momentarily cease movements during sexual activity. This may give your body the brief rest it needs to adjust.

7. Try diaphragmatic breathing through the sexual act. Breathe in as steadily as possible by consciously pulling your diaphragm down. What you are trying to avoid here are the short, panting breaths that may change the oxygen/carbon dioxide balance in your blood, thereby causing a headache.

8. Eliminate things that make you feel guilty. Specific environments, practices, or even contacts with particular individuals which may evoke feelings of guilt or embarrassment.

9

CHILDREN'S HEADACHES

Melissa Sherman was a vibrant, fun-loving nine-year-old, looking forward to her summer vacation. It wasn't that she hated school; it was just that the fourth grade had been so much harder for her than for the other kids in her class. Because of her headaches, she missed so many tests and assignments. Now her family was planning a special camping trip to Yellowstone National Park. She was so excited because she had never been there before. But Melissa was afraid her migraines might spoil the trip for her entire family. Her older brother and sister were already complaining that everything seemed to revolve around her "stupid" headaches. They seemed to think she used them just to get her way. It was so unfair. No one who had ever suffered through a migraine headache could think she made them happen on purpose.

The day of her fourth grade graduation was perfect, and her class party was great fun. Of course, she'd eaten a lot of things she wasn't supposed to, like a hot dog and two big slices of pepperoni pizza, but she'd felt OK. It wasn't until afterwards, when Melissa got home, that she began to feel sick. She noticed that her face was really pale and that she had dark circles under her eyes.

Melissa knew the signs. The headaches always seemed to start that way. Twice a month or so, she'd come home from school looking like that. And this time was no different. As the headache came on she grew increasingly irritable and went to her room. Turning off the lights she put her hands over her ears, trying to block out the normal household noises that suddenly seemed so maddeningly loud.

She tried to pretend that she was just tired—until her stomach began to hurt. The nausea came on so fast she barely made it to the bathroom in time to vomit. When she finally stopped throwing up, she was so tired she only had enough energy left to stumble back to her bed. She cried herself to sleep, afraid her migraine attack would spoil her family's plans to leave on their vacation in the morning.

For children like Melissa there will be many missed opportunities: the homecoming game in her sophomore year, playing in a soccer play-off, missing the first chance to take the SAT.

ONE OF MANY

Melissa is not alone. Unfortunately, headaches are a common complaint during childhood. More than half of those afflicted with adult migraine had their first attacks before they left their teens. Toddlers as young as three may suffer from childhood migraine. Some researchers have even found evidence that children may start having headaches as early as six weeks after birth.

Statistically speaking, 3 percent of those under seven get migraines, as do 5 percent of those between seven and twelve. Worse still, they afflict between 10 and 20 percent of all teenagers. The good news is that children who have migraines appear to have a better chance of growing out of them than adults. Almost half of all children who get migraines will stop having attacks at some point during their teenage years. Another quarter will cease getting migraines during their early adulthood.

But even so, a child's headache attacks are no less serious than an adult's and should never be overlooked. A headache is Mother Nature's way of telling parents that something is wrong with their child's body, food, or lifestyle. Parents must often intervene on their behalf and see that they get help.

Headache pain may signal a medical emergency, or it may indicate that a child feels unable to cope with a divorce or a problem at school. But whatever the underlying cause, headaches can lead to regressive or strange behavior, depression, withdrawal, and sleep and eating disorders. However, even though there are serious physical and emotional repercussions that can occur as a result of children's headaches, the vast majority of kids will never visit a pediatrician because parents are unaware of the potential dangers.

Migraine headaches in young people may follow the classical pattern, complete with accompanying aura and one-sided pain, but childhood migraine can affect both sides of the head. Children often suffer more frequent attacks, which are shorter in duration than those of adults. In some instances, the childhood migraine does not even persist into adulthood. But as with all migraine sufferers, in childhood and adolescent headache a family history of migraine is usually found.

Children with migraines often exhibit many of the same personality traits as adult sufferers, including anxiety, tension, and compulsive perfectionism. They also seem vulnerable to the same precipitating factors of diet , hunger, fatigue, and a change in routine that trigger adult migraines. Similarly, stressful or exciting events frequently set off a migraine attack in a susceptible teenager. Up until the age of puberty, boys and girls get migraine with equal frequency.

Tension-type headaches are not as common but do occur among children. As with adult tension headaches, the pain surrounds the head or forms a band around it and may involve neck tenderness and muscle spasms. And just like adults, children with a Type A personality seem to have a biochemical vulnerability to headaches. Because such kids tend to react more strongly to stress in family or school situations, they secrete more of the very adrenal hormones that are believed to initiate tension headaches. Minimizing or eliminating emotional stress may be all that is needed to bring the headache problem under control.

Despite myths to the contrary, children and teens feel pain as strongly as grown-ups. When a headache strikes, they suffer the same pounding head pain, nausea, vomiting, and aversion to light and sound that adults endure. Although a wide range of purely physical factors including fever, eyestrain, motion sickness, ear infections, measles and mumps can trigger headaches, hormones play a central role as well. The hormonal basis for migraine in children is thought to be much the same as in adults, involving the neurotransmitter hormones serotonin, adrenaline, and noradrenaline. But the symptoms of headache in children may be very different from those found in adults.

EARLY MIGRAINE SYMPTOMS

In childhood migraine, the aura phase may be characterized by dramatic neurological manifestations including confusion, listlessness, painful sensitivity to light, fever, hallucinations, dilated pupils, or difficulty speaking. In one form of childhood migraine known as basilar artery migraine, children may experience weakness or numbness on both sides of the body, vision problems, temporary balance problems, or dizziness during the aura phase. In basilar artery migraine, the blood vessels that feed the brain from the back of the neck and head can be constricted. The back of the brain is where the balance mechanisms are present.

Strangely enough, during the "headache" phase of an attack children with migraine may not experience head pain at all. They may suffer severe abdominal pain instead. Physicians call this phenomenon "abdominal migraine" or "migraine equivalent," and it may be compounded by motion sickness or recurrent bouts of nausea and vomiting that can last for several days. Abdominal migraine often develops into a more typical migraine headache pattern later in life. It is thought that the biliousness and colic found in some children may be early migraine symptoms.

Migraine equivalents other than abdominal pain include sudden mood changes, dizziness, blurred vision, unexplained fatigue, food cravings, nausea, or loss of appetite.

The variety of these symptoms may be explained partially by the fact that serotonin acts as both a neurotransmitter and a hormone. In this dual role it mediates many different body functions. When serotonin is initially released and then flushed from the body during the biochemical dysfunction that causes headache, a variety of other body functions may go awry as well. Serotonin is allegedly involved in the mechanism for hunger and sleep, for example, and certain maladies such as depression, anorexia nervosa, and obsessive-compulsive disorders.

Migraine attacks in children may also be marked by episodes of diarrhea and an elevated temperature of 102 or 103 degrees. This type of headache may understandably cause a good deal of alarm to parents when it first occurs. If your child experiences a similar attack every two or three months, however, your doctor should consider a diagnosis of migraine.

If you already know that your child suffers from migraines, be attentive if he or she becomes abruptly irritable, combative, or withdrawn, since mood changes often signal the hormonal changes that precipitate the aura, or pre-headache phase, of an attack. In light of the fact that about half of all childhood headaches develop upon waking or shortly afterward, you should be especially alert to grouchiness or complaints about physical discomfort at this time.

Difficulty in speaking or maintaining balance may also indicate that a child is experiencing the aura phase of migraine. He or she also may behave strangely and have trouble focusing the eyes. If you recognize these symptoms as the familiar warning signs of an impending headache, have your child lie down in a dark, quiet room and try to get him or her to relax and go to sleep. But if such symptoms are new to your child or more intense than usual, you should call your pediatrician for advice.

Because children, particularly young ones, may not be able to tell you what's wrong with them, it is up to you as a parent to observe your child's behavior for the warning signs of migraine.

TEENAGE HEADACHES

Even teenagers may not recognize or admit when they're starting to get a headache because they want so much to fit in and seem normal. Adolescence is a time of important life changes, when teenagers tend to experience troubled family lives, school difficulties, problems with friends, or sexual experimentation. Depression and stress-related headaches often follow such upheavals. As if that weren't enough, dieting, obesity, drug use, and the overconsumption of junk foods make teens even more vulnerable to headaches. That's why the percentage of teens who suffer from serious headaches is so high.

Of course, the female sex hormones estrogen and progesterone play a very important role in the frequency of headaches during adolescence. Up until the age of eleven, boys get more headaches than girls do. But all that changes between the ages of eleven and fourteen when girls begin to experience the hormonal shifts that start their menstrual cycles . These hormonal changes also trigger headaches, making young menstruating women far more susceptible to headache pain than teenage boys. In fact, in one recent study, 56 percent of boys and 74 percent of girls between the ages of twelve and seventeen reported having had headaches within the past month.

HEADACHES AND SCHOOL

It is not unusual for a doctor to examine a child with frequent and severe headaches that cause many absences from school. This type of headache often affects children between the ages of nine and fourteen. The headaches commonly occur on a daily basis, starting in the morning and continuing for two to three hours. Although it is sometimes difficult, a doctor must determine whether these headaches are tension headaches, migraine headaches, coexisting migraine and tension headaches, or an excuse to avoid school. In such cases parents must help their child understand that sickness is a problem to be dealt with, not a way to get attention or to avoid difficult tasks.

In the case of true migraine, the headache and therapy should be explained to a child, and he or she should be given clear instructions on how to deal with the headache. If children develop their headaches at school, their pain medication should be available, and their condition should be discussed with the teacher and the school nurse. It is very important that such children be encouraged to attend school and take appropriate measures to prevent the headache, whether by medication or diet.

A child's school years can determine whether or not he or she will live a productive and fulfilled life. When those years are devastated by recurrent headaches, children tend to fall behind academically, socially, and emotionally. Such children often personalize their illness. They see it as a punishment for bad behavior or as a sign that they're different or not as good as other children. These feelings can cause a child to become withdrawn, particularly when headaches force them to be absent from school a great deal.

The sudden, uncontrollable vomiting that commonly afflicts children during migraine attacks can also be embarrassing for them. Being away from the safety of their own home and the comforting familiarity of their family when such an attack occurs at school can be very frightening. This kind of episode singles a child out and makes him or her feel weird, different, weak, or sickly. As a result children can develop a strong aversion or phobia towards school after a severe migraine attack occurs there.

Their dread of another "school migraine" grows stronger every day until the stress can build high enough to bring on another attack. A vicious circle of pain-dread-pain can ensue. Parents can help break this circle by acknowledging their child's fears while helping to overcome them. Their goal should be to restore a child's sense of his or her own competence in school. Because this feeling of competence will decrease anxiety, headaches may strike less frequently. But a parent's main focus should center on restoring a child's inner motivation to go to school, whether or not the migraines continue to occur.

If your child has tension-type or coexisting migraine and tension-type headaches, you need to reassure him or her by letting the child know that a lot of people have them. A child's attitude toward his or her own migraine problem can be greatly improved by the knowledge that a favorite relative (maybe you) suffers with the same condition.

HEADACHE TREATMENT FOR CHILDREN

In treating children with migraine, doctors try to avoid the use of medications as much as possible, because they can have unpredictable effects on body systems that are still developing. In fact, headache drugs often have exaggerated side effects in children because of their smaller size and lower body weight. That's why it's best to start treatment with nothing stronger than aspirin or acetaminophen for pain relief (suppository and liquid forms are available for small children) and by teaching them behavioral pain management techniques like biofeedback and progressive muscle relaxation. Recent studies suggest that both techniques work equally well in children with chronic headaches.

Because they haven't yet developed a pain behavior pattern, children are very receptive to learning new "biophysical" techniques to relieve or block their headaches. And because they're not habituated to pain-killing drugs, they can actually use the biofeedback and relaxation techniques more fully than adults.

Biofeedback training is simply a way of learning how to control certain functions of the body by thought and will. Through biofeedback, for example, children can learn to slow their heart rates or lower their blood pressure.

Avoiding headache triggers is another important part of teaching children how to prevent headaches. The triggers for children's migraine and tension headache are the same ones that set off adult head pain. But every person is different. That means each child has his or her own set of triggers that first have to be identified before they can be avoided. To do that, it's a good idea to review possible headache triggers, such as disrupted sleep, environmental factors (such as secondhand smoke), unusual stress, or questionable foods, after every attack. For most children, as for many adults, sleep is the best solution once a headache actually strikes. It is important to stop children's headaches as soon as possible to prevent the headaches from becoming a lifelong problem. Discovering the headache trigger is vital. In this way, parents usually play an indispensable role in controlling their child's headache problem.

If these simple approaches don't provide relief, your doctor may want to cautiously try some of the drugs used to treat adult headaches. Like adults, children who get three or more serious headaches a month are usually eligible for preventive therapy. The search for an appropriate preventive might start with the drug cyproheptadine (Periactin) or the beta blocker propranolol.

Medications such as ergotamine tartrate and its derivatives are usually not prescribed for children unless the migraines are severe and persistent, as they have unpleasant side effects and must be used very carefully with young children.

AVOIDING HEADACHE TRIGGERS

Although people of all ages should eat a wholesome, well-balanced diet at regular meal times and follow a stable sleep schedule, it is especially important for children who suffer from chronic headaches. Unfortunately, children, especially teens, tend to have their own ideas about what constitutes a healthy lifestyle. All too often a piece of pizza or a hastily consumed hot dog takes the place of a meal. But that can spell almost certain trouble for a child or adolescent who suffers from chronic headaches.

It is vitally important for children and teenagers to become familiar with the specific agents or circumstances that can cause head pain. Once they do, they may be able to identify the trigger, or precipitating factor, that is setting off their headaches. Since many of these triggers can be avoided, learning to make informed choices about their diet and lifestyle is a simple way for children and teens to gain control of their headache problem. Many children, for example, are able to control their headaches once they learn to avoid foods that contain the amino acid, tyramine. (See chapter 11 for a description of common headache triggers.)

ACUTE HEADACHES

If a teenager gets a very painful headache with no history of similar headaches previously, an accurate diagnosis may save his or her life. Although the fever that strikes with the common flu can cause mild headaches, acutely painful headaches accompanied by fever may signal a dangerous disorder like meningitis or encephalitis.

And as with adults, headaches that get progressively more severe, increase with movement, or wake a child from sleep may warn of a brain tumor. Although such cases are rare, accompanying neurological symptoms like blurred vision, balance problems, weakness, lethargy, and personality change are clear danger signals that should never be ignored.

If a child experiences seizures and headaches, the patient requires an urgent neurological workup.

10

DRUGS TO PREVENT AND TREAT HEADACHES

Mattie's headaches started when she was eighteen and initially occurred only during her menstrual period. During college, these headaches with the ergot suppository given to her by her doctor. The first few years after graduation from Howard University, Mattie did remarkably well with her headaches. She moved to Chicago to live with her older sister and taught in the Chicago public schools while attending graduate school. She married a Chicago policeman after obtaining her master's degree in education and continued to teach after her two sons were born.

The headaches, which had disappeared with each pregnancy, started to increase after she began taking birth control pills. Mattie stopped the Pill, but the migraine headaches continued to occur every one to two weeks. And then her life was almost shattered when her husband was killed responding to a burglar alarm. Mattie was faced with raising their two young sons, ages eight and eleven, by herself. She also realized that the household income would be seriously decreased. She asked her widowed mother to live with her to help with the child rearing. Then Mattie returned to graduate school to obtain a Ph.D. in school administration.

When Mattie first consulted me she was finishing her doctoral dissertation and breathing a sigh of relief that her oldest son had been accepted to West Point. Raising the boys in a neighborhood that bordered a gang area had been very challenging, and she had confronted the problem courageously. But her headaches had continued to increase and were beginning to impact on her life. When she wasn't suffering from a severe migraine attack one to two times a week she was struggling to cope with the pain of a chronic tension headache every day. Mattie complained of a sleep disturbance in that she woke up several times a night and then had difficulty falling back to sleep.

She had tried numerous headache medications with minimal success. For the severe migraine headaches she was taking an ergot suppository every day, and she had noticed that if she skipped the suppository, which she usually inserted before leaving her job as a school principal, she would get a bad headache. For the milder headaches, she was using over-the-counter analgesics that contain caffeine. I have a standard question for my new patients: How long does a bottle of 100 aspirin (or acetaminophen or ibuprofen) last you? Mattie told me that a bottle would last her about ten days.

Mattie's history underscored the need for admission to a specialized inpatient headache unit. Mattie was suffering from coexisting migraine and tension-type headaches. She was also experiencing two types of rebound phenomena due to excessive ergot and caffeine overuse. When ergot is taken on a daily basis the patient develops an increasing tolerance to this drug. If she misses a dose of the ergot she'll experience a rebound headache. My patients are always instructed to maintain a four-day interval between uses of ergot drugs. Mattie was also suffering caffeine-rebound headaches. On a daily basis, she was taking upwards of eight to ten tablets of a caffeine-containing analgesic. It was important for us to wean Mattie completely off the ergot agent as well as the caffeine-containing analgesic.

To withdraw Mattie from these drugs she was admitted to our inpatient unit. There Mattie received injections of a sedative with antinauseant effects. This type of therapy helped her deal with the severe headaches that develop from the withdrawal. Upon discharge she was taught how to inject herself with sumatriptan to abort the migraine headache. For the daily headache Mattie was given a NSAID, ketorolac (Toradol), to be used whenever she experienced pain. Ketorolac is probably a more effective pain manager than any of the other oral NSAIDs.

Before admission Mattie had been treated with a calcium channel blocker for hypertension. Because this group of drugs is also being used for migraine, I discussed Mattie's case with her internist, who agreed that she could be changed to a different calcium channel blocker, verapamil, which has been more effective in migraine preventive therapy. When Mattie was admitted to the inpatient unit she was also started on preventive therapy. We have found that treatment of coexisting migraine and tension-type headaches is complex because of the two types of headaches present. Antidepressants have been particularly helpful in treating both types of these headaches.

Because Mattie had a personal and family history of increased eye pressure, glaucoma, I had to consult with her ophthalmologist before initiating treatment. Glaucoma is a disease of the eye that is evidenced by increased eye pressure and a decrease in the field of vision. The tricyclic antidepressants that are used frequently in the treatment of coexisting migraine and tension-type headache are contraindicated in patients with closed-angle glaucoma. That is why I opted, with her ophthalmologist's consent, to start Mattie on a newer antidepressant, fluoxetine (Prozac).

During hospitalization Mattie participated in many of the activities organized on the unit and also received biofeedback training. Despite her long history of headache and dependency on analgesics, Mattie became enthusiastic about learning the biofeedback techniques (Biofeedback will be explained in detail in chapter 11). She also enjoyed classes in art therapy, relaxation training, and diet. Although her headaches had only decreased minimally, she felt she had made some important gains in her recovery and had also learned a great deal about her headache problem. Eventually Mattie was put on a monoamine oxidase inhibitor (MAOI), and this combination therapy finally did the trick for her.

WHICH DRUG IS RIGHT FOR YOU?

The treatment of headache can be divided into four main categories: general treatment measures, abortive therapy, preventive therapy, and pain relief. Selecting which type or how many types of therapies depends on the type of headache you experience. For episodic headache, those headaches occurring fewer than three times per month, preventive therapy would not be indicated. However, preventive therapy is indicated for those patients experiencing chronic tension-type headache, more than two migraines per month, or acute cluster headaches.

GENERAL TREATMENT MEASURES

Increased gains in headache research have produced a greater quantity of drugs available for both abortive and preventive therapy. Your treatment regimen will depend on your diagnosis. The important facets of general treatment measures are identification and avoidance of headache triggers. Headache triggers are described in further detail in chapter 11. General treatment measures include diet and maintaining strict sleeping and meal schedules, as well as coping strategies. We all recognize that stress is impossible to avoid, but if the patient can learn to handle stress through relaxation methods and coping strategies, she may be able to prevent headaches related to stress. Progressive relaxation and breathing exercises, included in chapter 11, are also useful in regards to general treatment measures. Biofeedback therapy, because it is a nondrug treatment, is included in general treatment measures.

ABORTIVE THERAPY

The key to abortive therapy is using it as early as possible in an acute attack. For many years ergotamine tartrate was the agent of choice in the prevention of migraine.

Ergotamine Tartrate: Ergotamine works by causing the muscular layer of the blood vessels to constrict. Ergotamine should be taken as early as possible in a migraine attack in order to be effective. The only forms of ergotamine available in the United States are in combination products with caffeine. Caffeine acts to potentiate or synergize ergotamine, which is why it is added to ergotamine. These agents are available as oral tablets or as rectal suppositories. Before prescribing which ergotamine is to be used, the physician must consider the environment and the time at which the patient usually gets the migraine attacks. An ergotamine derivative, dihydroergotamine mesylate (DHE) is available at this time only as an injection. Many patients are taught self-injection techniques so that they can use DHE at the first sign of a headache. As stated earlier in Mattie's case, patients receiving an ergotamine must include a four-day interval between days of use of the drug. Ergotamine agents and DHE should not be used if you have cardiac or circulatory problems as they can cause a decrease in the circulation of blood in the hands and legs.

Isometheptene Mucate: I find isometheptene mucate (Midrin) to be one of the most helpful drugs for people who are not able to take the ergot preparations or who prefer not to take such a powerful drug. This drug is also welcomed by patients whose headaches are easily amenable to less heroic forms of relief. Isometheptene mucate has vasoconstrictor effects similar to ergotamine but without the adverse effects. In Midrin, it is combined with dichloralphenazone and acetaminophen, which offers relief from the associated symptoms of a migraine attack, including nausea and vomiting.

Sumatriptan: Sumatriptan (Imitrex) represents the very latest in migraine relief. In the U.S. it is available for administration only by injection. Given as a subcutaneous (under the skin) injection, sumatriptan has stopped acute migraine attacks in the majority of the patients tested. Most people begin to feel relief in about twenty minutes after an injection of sumatriptan, and their headaches completely disappear within one to two hours. One of sumatriptan's advantages over other drugs is that its side effects are far less severe and less frequent. These side effects can include dizziness, tingling, sensations of warmth, and pressure-like sensations in the chest.

How does it work? Scientists aren't completely sure, but the new drug appears to mimic some of the beneficial actions of serotonin, at the same time helping block serotonin's inflammatory effects. Serotonin, you remember, is a powerful yet mysterious hormone given off by the platelets in the blood stream. In the initial warning phase of migraine attacks serotonin tells the blood vessels around the brain to constrict so less blood and oxygen gets through. This causes the visual warning symptoms or aura. But then it inexplicably directs the blood vessels to stop constricting and begins to dilate their walls instead.

Sumatriptan should not be used in patients with previous cardiac problems or angina or by those patients with uncontrolled hypertension. Sumatriptan is never used jointly with ergotamine, and as with all drugs, should not be used during pregnancy.

NSAIDs: Today the treatment of choice for the prevention of menstrual headaches is a new group of pain-relieving (analgesic) drugs related to aspirin. Aspirin was the first of these nonsteroidal anti-inflammatory drugs, known as NSAIDs. The NSAIDs, including aspirin, interrupt the pain cycle by blocking the production of pain-producing prostaglandins and act as anti-inflammatory agents. But they also curtail the platelet clumping that triggers serotonin release. Although aspirin is very effective at relieving many types of headaches, it often doesn't stop migraine pain. Other NSAIDs are more powerful and more selective in their activity against migraine, particularly naproxen sodium (Anaprox). For the preventive treatment of menstrual migraine, the NSAIDs have demonstrated great success.

The NSAIDs used in menstrual migraine include naproxen sodium (Anaprox), fenoprofen calcium (Nalfon), naproxen (Naprosyn), ketoprofen (Orudis), and nabumetone

(Relafen). These drugs should be taken two to three days before the menstrual flow begins and continued through the flow. NSAIDs are particularly useful because they not only block prostaglandin production, but they also prevent platelet aggregation and swelling as well. Ibuprofen in non-prescription doses is now available over the counter as is naproxen sodium. Both of these drugs do work but in larger doses than are available in over-the-counter products. These drugs are typically effective in larger doses, but you should discuss the doses with your physician.

Since the new breed of NSAIDs are more powerful painkillers than aspirin, they can be used in lower doses; this produces fewer side effects. Ketorolac is an NSAID that is available in both oral and injectable forms. The introduction of the injectable form has provided an excellent alternative to narcotic analgesics. Its actions are similar to other NSAIDs, but it does not have the potential risk of drug habituation associated with narcotics.

Like their therapeutic effects, the side effects of the NSAIDs are similar. These drugs prevent or quell headache pain by reducing the overproduction of prostaglandins in the cranial arteries. Such side effects could include gastrointestinal inflammation and liver damage. Asthma attacks, severe skin rashes, and even headache might follow NSAID use in the rare cases of patients who are allergic to it. If an adverse reaction results from using one NSAID drug, there is a higher risk of a similar reaction from other members of the NSAID group. If necessary, a trial with low doses of each of the NSAIDs can be tried, elevating dosages gradually if the patient suffers no side effects. Most of the severe side effects of NSAID therapy only trouble patients who take large quantities of them daily for arthritis. In the smaller amounts used to treat menstrual headaches, the incidence of side effects is much lower.

Patients should also be aware that NSAIDs can react with other drugs, largely because the NSAIDs slow the liver's ability to metabolize other drugs and hinder the kidneys' abilities to excrete them. Make sure your doctor knows about any drug, even an over-the-counter one, that you are currently taking. Patients who are currently taking the drug warfarin (Coumadin), which is used for patients recovering from a stroke or cardiac problems, should be especially careful. Because all the NSAIDs inhibit clotting, they should not be given to anyone with a bleeding disorder.

But despite the adverse effects that occasionally occur with the use of NSAIDs, most physicians consider these drugs to be as safe as aspirin. And because many women who suffer from menstrual headaches do not respond to standard headache drugs, the NSAIDs have proven to be a welcome breakthrough in the treatment of such headaches.

PREVENTIVE MEASURES

As we stated previously, preventive treatment must be considered if the patient is suffering two or more migraines per month or if the headaches are of such severity that they seriously impact the patient's daily life. In cluster headache, because of the short duration of the attacks, abortive and pain-relieving measures have to be used too frequently, and the patient is in need of preventive therapy in order to stop the cycle of headaches.

Beta Blockers: The agents of choice in migraine prevention treatment are the beta blockers. The introduction of beta blockers into migraine-prevention treatment was an accident. These drugs were originally used for hypertension and cardiac arrhythmia problems. A patient using propranolol (Inderal) for hypertension noted that during treatment she did not experience any migraine headaches. This finding led to investigations into the use of beta blockers in migraine therapy, with the results looking very promising. Propranolol was the first beta blocker approved by the Food and Drug Administration for migraine prevention. Timolol (Blocadren) is the second beta blocker approved for migraine treatment.

Beta blockers work in migraine prevention in two ways. First, beta blockers prevent platelet clumping which in turn prevents serotonin release. Second, they block the dilation of the cranial arteries. Propranolol cannot be used in patients with asthma, congestive heart failure, or chronic obstructive lung disease. For these patients, we can use other beta blockers called cardioselective, which are suitable for patients with respiratory problems. Metoprolol (Lopressor) is a cardioselective beta blocker that is approved by the FDA for treatment of hypertension but not as yet for migraine.

Alpha Agonists: The use of alpha agonists in the treatment of migraines was also discovered by accident. These drugs were originally used successfully in the treatment of hypertension. Like the beta blockers, these drugs are effective due to their action on the blood vessels. They differ from the beta blockers in their chemical configuration. The alpha agonist most often used is clonidine (Catapres). Clonidine has not achieved popular application in the U.S. but has been recognized in Europe as effective for those patients whose migraine attacks are especially associated with tyramine-containing foods. Tyramine is considered a trigger of migraine attacks.

Calcium Channel Blockers: Calcium channel blockers have been used for heart disease and in treating patients recovering from stroke. These drugs act by blocking the release of serotonin and regulating the ionic calcium, thus controlling the blood vessels' expansion and contraction. This action stabilizes the blood vessels and prevents the headache. These drugs are used in migraine treatment because of the vascular nature of migraine. The calcium channel blockers that have been used effectively in migraine include nimodipine (Nimotop) and verapamil (Calan, Isoptin, Verelan). Because these drugs have not yet received approval for use in migraine, research continues into their role in migraine therapy. Verapamil, in particular, is noted for its long-term effects in decreasing the frequency, severity, and duration of migraine. With verapamil, the most commonly reported side effect is constipation. Other calcium channel blockers such as diltiazem (Cardizem) and nifedipine (Procardia) have not shown significant results in migraine.

Antidepressants: As discussed in earlier chapters, antidepressants also play a role in headache prevention by affecting serotonin receptors. Antidepressants have been investigated for well over thirty years for their role in migraine prevention. Their effective use in the treatment of chronic tension-type headaches due to depression is well documented.

A list of currently available antidepressants continues to grow and includes amitriptyline (Elavil, Endep), doxepin (Sinequan), nortriptyline (Pamelor), desipramine (Norpramin), imipramine (Tofranil), trimipramine (Surmontil), amoxapine (Asendin), trazodone (Desyrel), fluoxetine (Prozac), bupropion (Wellbutrin), maprotiline (Ludiomil), sertaline (Zoloft), paroxetine (Paxil), and venlafaxine (Effexor).

NSAIDs: The nonsteroidal anti-inflammatories have also been used successfully in migraine prevention probably due to their effects on both the prostaglandins and their anti-inflammatory effects. The NSAIDs that have been used effectively in migraine prevention include naproxen, aspirin, ketoprofen, tolmetin sodium, and fenoprofen calcium.

Platelet Antagonists: All NSAIDs, including aspirin, are platelet antagonists. As discussed earlier, during a migraine attack blood platelets will clump together and begin releasing serotonin, which causes the blood vessels to dilate or expand. Accordingly, a drug that could act on the platelets and prevent these actions would probably be beneficial in thwarting a migraine attack.

Aspirin was the first of these platelet antagonists. Although aspirin has long been used for pain relief, it is now coming into its own as a preventive medicine. In a study of more than 20,000 physicians who used aspirin on a daily basis, many were migraine sufferers who noted that their headaches had significantly decreased while using the daily medication. Investigations are currently under way to see if daily aspirin intake will be effective for female migraine sufferers.

Other platelet antagonists are sulfinpyrazone and dipridamole. These drugs have been marginally effective for preventing migraine attacks but have not gained widespread use.

Methysergide: The only other agent approved for migraine prevention other than the beta blockers, propranolol and timolol, is methysergide (Sansert). This drug is closely related to the ergot alkaloids. Its effectiveness in migraine therapy is identified with its anti-inflammatory and vasoconstrictor effects. Despite its successful use, long-term therapy with methysergide is associated with severe side effects. Because of the potential for these harmful effects, methysergide is not used frequently in migraine. A patient on methysergide for a continuous treatment period of six months must undergo a four- to six-week break from the drug. Due to the self-limiting nature of cluster headache, methysergide is the drug of choice in treating cluster headache as the patients will not require long treatment. Methysergide should never be used in patients with a history of ulcer disease, phlebitis, severe hypertension, or pulmonary disease.

Cyproheptadine: For children with migraine, cyproheptadine (Periactin) is an antihistamine that has been used successfully. It has not shown the same effectiveness in adults with migraine. Its low side-effect profile, except for weight gain, is welcomed by those physicians treating children with headaches.

PAIN RELIEVING MEASURES

Unfortunately, patients may not find complete relief from the attack with abortive agents, and analgesics will be needed. The agents available as over-the-counter analgesics include aspirin, acetaminophen, ibuprofen, and naproxen sodium. As in Mattie's case, there is always a danger of over-consumption of the analgesics, particularly those containing caffeine. As we stated, withdrawal from the caffeine-containing agents may trigger the caffeine-withdrawal headache. Other pain relieving measures are available, such as the narcotic analgesics, which must be prescribed by your physician. Frequent use of these analgesics must be avoided to prevent dependency.

The antiemetic drugs used to prevent nausea and vomiting, which are typically associated symptoms of migraine, are often used as pain-relieving measures and include the phenothiazines. Some of these agents are used because they have a sedative action. Phenothiazines include promethazine (Phenergan), chlorpromazine (Thorazine), and prochlorperazine (Compazine). For those patients who do not need a sedative effect, other antiemetics such as trimethobenzamide (Tigan) and metoclopramide (Reglan) may also be used.

Butorphanol: Butorphanol (Stadol) is a synthetic narcotic analgesic that has been used for many years as an injectable medication. It is now available as a nasal spray, which speeds up the action of the drug and decreases the risk associated with the injections. Butorphanol is especially effective for headache if the patient has not responded to abortive agents. It must be used discriminately because there is a small potential for dependency.

STATUS MIGRAINE

Some unfortunate patients will experience migraine that lasts more than twenty-four hours. This is believed to be due to an inflammation around the blood vessels, which are enlarged. Two forms of therapies are used for these headaches, corticosteroids and DHE. The corticosteroids are used because of their effects on inflammation. The patient may receive an injection of long-acting dexamethasone or may receive the oral tablets for a defined treatment period such as two to three days. Some researchers have found that DHE used with metoclopramide, an antinauseant, is effective in treating status migraine. Investigations continue into the therapy of status migraine.

WHEN YOUR MEDICATION
STOPS WORKING

Severe migraines are so painful that the threat of their return kindles fear in even the most valiant. At the slightest hint of oncoming pain, you run for the medicine cabinet and take whatever has proven effective in the past. But frequently, overuse or chronic use of medicines, both prescription and nonprescription, can cause their effectiveness to diminish. When you increase your dosage, it may be no more effective, but you experience more of the negative side effects. It's not fair, but unfortunately, this is one of the costs of a chronic illness like migraine.

Why does it happen? Your body can develop either resistance or a tolerance for the drug you've found effective in the past. In either case bigger doses don't mean more pain relief. That's why I always ask new patients how long a bottle of aspirin, for example, lasts them. If they're using it up too quickly, it's a good indication that they have developed a resistance or tolerance to the drugs they are using.

What to do? When your medicine begins to lose its effectiveness, return to your doctor. Ask him or her to prescribe something else. With numerous medications at our disposal, no one needs to suffer the pain of migraine any more. Take my advice. It's just not worth fighting. If you think your medications are less effective than they used to be, see your doctor.

IF YOU'RE PREGNANT

As we discussed in chapter 5, if you're pregnant, I don't recommend the use of any pharmacologic agents (drugs) in the first three months of pregnancy. If you become pregnant or plan on becoming pregnant in the near future, talk to your physician immediately. There are nondrug alternatives, which we'll discuss in the next chapter.

11

How to Help Yourself

When Paige Randolph first visited our clinic, I was struck by her cool beauty, effectively handling the fact that she was in the middle of a migraine attack. As soon as she removed her sunglasses, however, her eyes betrayed her pain. Even the dim halogen light in the examining room increased her suffering. While she was waiting, she had been forced to ask the nurse if she could leave the room if she felt she had to vomit. In spite of the pain she was able to provide a detailed history, which was typical of migraine with aura, with a previous menstrual relationship.

Her first memory of headache had been at the age of fourteen, while she was at a finishing school in Virginia. Since she remembered her aunt and grandmother having headaches, Paige took these migraine attacks as a matter of course. In addition to her grandmother's classic beauty and antebellum estate, Paige had inherited her tendency for migraine. Over the years she had tried to learn how to control these headaches and not let the headaches control her.

By the time Paige visited the Diamond Headache Clinic she had a thirty-five-year history of recurrent migraine attacks. They usually occurred with her periods, but they struck at other times during the month as well. The headaches had disappeared during her four pregnancies but had returned after a hysterectomy at age forty. She often noticed that her headaches appeared after a stressful event, such as the morning after her oldest daughter's wedding.

Paige had married shortly after graduating from college. She became pregnant with Allison while on her honeymoon, and she had to learn to become a homemaker and mother before her twenty-third birthday. Her husband joined a prestigious law firm in Charleston, and Paige had quickly adopted the role of young socialite, working tirelessly for charity and social causes.

Part of Paige's problem was that she could not say "no." In the same month she would chair a fashion show for a local school and also head a decorations committee for a hospital benefit. Paige, like many migraine sufferers, just took on too much. After finishing a project she would need two to three days to recover from the inevitable migraine that followed.

Her husband bragged about the perfect hostess he had married and the impeccable housekeeper she had become. Paige was proud of her perfect image and strove to maintain it. On several occasions when a migraine would hit after a dinner party, Paige would be washing the dishes on one side of the sink and vomiting into the other side.

Paige consulted her gynecologist for the migraine attacks. She was given an ergotamine suppository to use at the first sign of the headache, usually when she experienced the aura. This seemed to work at first, but when she received treatment for varicose veins, the legacy of four pregnancies, the gynecologist and internist appropriately discontinued the ergotamine, and the headaches returned.

Paige's younger daughter, Jordan, had become my patient, as she was attending Northwestern University in nearby Evanston. Jordan had responded very well to the use of sumatriptan to prevent her migraine attacks and had been particularly successful on biofeedback training. She advised her mother about this nondrug treatment, and Paige was curious.

Jordan accompanied her mother on that first visit and asked me to take special care of her. Because Paige's medical history was typical of migraine with aura, I was confident that we could find a solution to her problem. The headaches were occurring two to three times per month, and I believed that she would respond well to prophylactic therapy and recommended a trial on a daily dose of propranolol.

But Paige Randolph would have nothing to do with my recommendation. "I have no intention of taking medicine every day for a headache that comes two or three times per month."

I asked if she would consider using the sumatriptan when she was experiencing a severe headache. "Yes," she said, "and you may as well start with the one I have coming on right now." The nurse gave Paige an injection of sumatriptan and waited until she was feeling better to instruct her on self-injection techniques.

Before I left the exam room, Paige stopped me and said she was interested in our biofeedback training program. Although she was not a candidate for hospitalization, I did recommend that she schedule a two-week intensive biofeedback course at the Clinic. The always enthusiastic Paige wanted to start that day. That afternoon Paige began training

on both muscle relaxation and temperature-training biofeedback.

NONDRUG THERAPIES

For those whose headaches seem resistant to standard medical care, a wide variety of self-help techniques and treatments are available. Some are new, like biofeedback. Others
are ancient, like acupuncture. Still others use techniques for
relaxation and mind-over-body control that are based on
yoga. Although the value of these treatments continues to be
debated, all seem to work on some headaches for some people some of the time.

First, a word of caution. Many of these treatments are
offered by specialists who, though they may be skilled in
their specialty, have a vested interest in treating the patient
in this manner to the exclusion of other forms of therapy
that may be more appropriate. Your best bet for headaches
that have resisted standard therapy is a headache clinic,
where a variety of experts from diverse fields can offer a
multipronged approach. In the long run, you'll usually save
time, frustration, and money—not to mention the fact that
you'll surely get at least some degree of relief. Many
headache clinics, such as ours in Chicago, offer many of these
alternative approaches.

The first headache clinic was created just after World
War II. In 1945 doctors at the Montefiore Hospital and
Medical Center in New York created a special department to
treat the growing number of clinic patients suffering from all
sorts of headache problems. Our clinic, the Diamond
Headache Clinic in Chicago, is the oldest privately owned
clinic in the country. In this country, especially in the past
few years, alternative approaches have gained wide accep-
tance by specialists in the field of headache pain.

BIOFEEDBACK

Biofeedback is probably the most effective of the mind-over-body techniques available. But it falls into a broader category of treatment known as behavior modification. So let's take a look at its roots, which are firmly fixed in the scientific method.

In behavior modification, you can learn to control either your external actions or habits, or your internal conscious or unconscious bodily functions. In medicine, the idea is that you exert your conscious control in order to produce a health benefit. In the case of headaches, you can learn to relax the muscles of your head, neck, and upper back, which are responsible for muscle-tension headaches, or you can even learn to control the blood flow in the vessels both inside and outside your skull to relieve the pain of migraines.

One of the conscious behaviors you can learn to control is your reaction to stress. Many chronic headaches are either partially or entirely stress induced. Researchers have found that reducing your reaction to stress through behavior modification often helps avoid headaches.

Many behavior modification techniques are based on the ancient Oriental systems of yoga and Zen Buddhism. That doesn't mean you must take part in certain religious practices, however, to gain some benefit from the thousands of years of practical experience that these systems have compiled.

The concept that the mind can gain control over previously unconscious functions of the body was long scoffed at by Western medicine, though it's been studied in the West since at least the turn of the century. In 1901, a psychologist named Joseph H. Bair attached electrodes to a muscle above the ears of student volunteers and instructed them to press a button wired to deliver a mild electrical charge. The charge caused their ears to wiggle. Of course, this was the source of great hilarity in the classroom until Bair revealed the practical aspect of the exercise. He asked his students to then try to learn to wiggle their ears on their own, without the electric shocks.

At first the students tried grimacing, brow furrowing, and jaw clenching in their comical attempts to duplicate the wiggling ears. Slowly they were able to focus on the specific muscles involved and eventually were successful.

The experiment was just a curiosity for many years until the concept surfaced in Germany in the 1920s. A Berlin psychiatrist named Johannes Schultz developed a self-hypnosis-like technique he called autogenic training. He taught his patients that by repeating affirmative statements they could relax and lower their pulse rate and blood pressure. Patients were instructed to close their eyes and repeat to themselves, "My arms and legs are heavy. My arms and legs are warm. My heartbeat is calm and regular. My breathing is relaxed and comfortable."

Dr. Schultz found that after a few months' practice his patients could increase the skin temperature of their hands and feet by one or two degrees. This temperature increase indicated that blood vessels in the patients' hands and feet were dilating and more blood was flowing to them. This in turn lowered their blood pressure and pulse rate by 10 percent. In addition, he found that breathing and brain-wave activity also slowed. As a result, stress-related afflictions, such as sleeplessness, ulcers, and headache, were improved in his patients.

At about the same time in the U.S., Dr. Edmund Jacobson of the University of Chicago began experimenting with a technique that would later be called progressive relaxation. In this simple approach, a patient is asked to tense a target muscle and really feel the tension in that muscle. Then the patient is asked to fully relax it. Gradually the patient learns to recognize small changes in muscle tension and relaxation.

Next, Dr. Jacobson told his subjects to pretend in their minds that they were operating an old-fashioned telegraph key with their middle finger—but not to move their finger. He found that the muscles of the middle finger were being bombarded with the same nerve impulses one would expect during normal movement.

What was happening? His patients were selectively bypassing parts of the nervous system. Dr. Jacobson went on to prove that anxiety can be the result of people's muscles becoming tense just from imagining a stressful situation. In other words, worrying makes your muscles tense.

Today that doesn't really seem too far-fetched, but the concept has important ramifications for headache control. We now know that with practice, regular use of progressive relaxation can prevent headaches in some patients.

During the 1960s the use of biofeedback in medicine was found serendipitously. Researcher Elmer Green of the Menninger Clinic in Topeka, Kansas, had studied the effects of yoga and the yogis' ability to unconsciously control certain physical functions such as their pulse rate and blood pressure. In order to investigate these techniques, Dr. Green and his staff used electronic instruments that measured these physiologic functions. He noted that one volunteer incurred a severe migraine when her hand temperature decreased. When her headache disappeared, the hand temperature elevated. Using these findings, Dr. Green and his staff further investigated the use of these instruments in treating migraine patients to get rid of their acute attacks. By using imagery and relaxation, the patient would attempt to increase hand temperature. A temperature-measuring device was placed on the dominant index finger to record any changes. They were very successful in this research and Dr. Green proposed a "hot hands" theory for treating migraine.

Temperature training is now used extensively in headache treatment. Through temperature training, the patient focuses on warming the hand and thereby redirecting blood flow into the hand. The use of autogenic phrases focuses more on relaxation while the patient is attached to the thermometer. Patients may focus on warm images such as sitting by a fire, by a beach, or drinking a hot cup of tea. By using these techniques at the first sign of a headache the patient may be able to abort the acute attack. We also recommend that the patient continue to practice these techniques to maintain their skills.

In biofeedback, sensitive electronic instruments amplify subtle changes in biological functions and display them for the test subjects so they can attempt to influence them with their conscious will. Temperature regulation, heartbeat, respiration, muscle contraction, and brain-wave activity can all be monitored, and the results immediately returned to the patient by a variety of audio or visual methods. Brain-wave activity is frequently monitored by a series of audio tones: higher tones for normal awake states and lower tones for the deeper levels of relaxation. Skin temperature can be monitored by a patient simply watching a sensitive digital thermometer.

MUSCLE-RELAXATION BIOFEEDBACK

We know that much of the pain in tension-type headaches is caused by a tightening of the muscles of the neck and in and around the head. Although the hormonal shifts of a woman's menstrual cycle aren't directly involved with triggering tension-type headaches, other hormones may be the root of the cause. Biofeedback, however, can help both migraine and tension-type headaches even if they're hormonally related. Through biofeedback, patients can be taught to relax those muscles, and by relaxing them to reduce or eliminate their pain. The technique is particularly helpful to combat stress, which is a major headache trigger. Stress causes the adrenal glands to pump out the hormone adrenaline, which narrows blood vessels and brings on headaches. Since stress does far more harm to the body than just cause headaches, learning to relax through biofeedback could be considered a vital link to health.

At our clinic we bring the patient into a quiet, dimly lit room and have her sit in a comfortable chair or lie down on a couch. The patient puts on earphones and has four electrical pickups taped to the frontalis muscle across the forehead. Generally, when the frontalis muscle relaxes, we find that so do the muscles of the scalp, neck, and upper body.

The electrodes are connected to an instrument that converts the tension in the muscle into a particular kind of sound. As long as the frontalis muscle is contracted or is under great tension, a high whining sound is heard. The more tense the frontalis muscle becomes, the higher pitched is the tone that the patient hears. When the frontalis muscle starts relaxing, the sound lowers both in tone and volume.

Since the lower tone is more pleasant and since it can be achieved by relaxing the frontalis muscle, the patient soon learns to relax that muscle and by doing so to relax the muscles of the scalp, neck, shoulders, and upper back. The sound of the tone is a signal to the patient of how tense the muscles are. By responding to that tone, she learns where her muscles are and how to relax them individually. But that's not all there is to it. We've found that progressive relaxation

exercises are helpful, particularly if practiced on a daily basis.
Here is an example of what a trainer might tell you to learn
to say to yourself:

> *Let all your muscles go loose and heavy. Just settle back quietly
> and comfortably. Wrinkle up your forehead now. Wrinkle and
> smooth it out. Picture the entire forehead and scalp becoming
> smoother as the relaxation increases. Now frown and crease
> your brows and study the tension. Let go of the tension.
> Smooth out the forehead once more. Now close your eyes
> tighter and tighter. Feel the tension. Now relax your eyes. Keep
> your eyes closed, gently, comfortably, and notice the relax-
> ation. Now clench your jaws. Bite your teeth together. Study
> the tension throughout the jaws. Relax your jaws now. Let
> your lips part slightly. Appreciate the relaxation.*
>
> *Now press your tongue hard against the roof of your
> mouth. All right, let your tongue return to a comfortable and
> relaxed position. Now purse your lips. Press your lips together
> tighter and tighter. Now relax your lips. Note the contrast
> between tension and relaxation. Feel the relaxation all over
> your face, all over your forehead and scalp, all over your eyes,
> jaws, lips, tongue, and your neck muscles. Press your head
> back as far as it can go and feel the tension in the neck. Roll
> it to the right and feel the tension shift. Now roll it to the left.
> Straighten your head and bring it forward and press your
> chin against your chest. Let your head return to a comfortable
> position, and study the relaxation. Let the relaxation develop.*
>
> *Shrug your shoulders. Right straight up. Hold the tension.
> Drop your shoulders and feel the relaxation. Feel how relaxed
> your neck and shoulders are. Shrug your shoulders again and
> move them around. Feel the tension in your shoulders and in
> your upper back. Drop your shoulders, right into your back
> muscles. Relax your neck and throat and your jaws and other
> facial areas as the pure relaxation takes over and grows deeper,
> deeper, ever deeper.*

After several periods of practice, perhaps a week or two,
you are able to relax the key muscles. Simply exercise your

ability to relax your muscles and in doing so reduce the pain the taut muscles were causing.

While practicing biofeedback, remember, DO NOT TRY TOO HARD. Relaxation is passive. You should not try to force your responses, but rather allow them to happen. The more you practice biofeedback, the more you will become aware of and be able to change your physiological responses to stress.

There's no doubt about it, biofeedback is quite simply one of the best methods for treating migraine and tension headaches. With this technique we can train people to control previously unused or involuntary bodily functions. Biofeedback actually enables a person to gain conscious control of her blood pressure, brain-wave activity, and blood flow to different parts of the body.

TEMPERATURE BIOFEEDBACK

In temperature biofeedback training patients attempt to learn how to increase the blood flow through their hands by watching meters that register the temperature in their fingertips. As the flow of blood into and through their hands increases, fingertip temperatures increase.

You begin by "thinking relaxation."

"I feel quiet. . . . I am beginning to feel quite relaxed," you start out saying to yourself.

> *My feet feel heavy and relaxed. . . . My ankles, my knees, and my hips feel heavy, relaxed, and comfortable. . . . My solar plexus and the whole central portion of my body feel relaxed and quiet. . . . My hands, my arms, and my shoulders feel heavy, relaxed, and comfortable. . . . My neck, my jaws, and my forehead feel relaxed. . . . They feel comfortable and smooth. . . . My whole body feels quiet, heavy, comfortable, and relaxed.*

Then you gradually shift the focus of your thinking from relaxation to increasing the temperature of your hands, as they feel warm, then warmer, then hot.

> *I am quite relaxed. . . . My arms and hands are heavy and warm. . . . I feel quiet. . . . My whole body is relaxed, and my hands are warm, relaxed, and warm. . . . My hands are warm. . . . Warmth is flowing into my hands. . . . They are warm . . . warmer . . . even warmer now.*

Some individuals think about their hands being immersed in a bucket of increasingly hot water.

The idea is that thinking about the hands growing hot will, under biofeedback theory, increase the flow of blood to and through the hands. By increasing blood volume in the hands the blood volume in the head will decrease, and this in turn will decrease the pressure on painfully swollen blood vessels of a tension-type headache or the last stage of a migraine.

Once patients learn to apply the sensors, Temperature Biofeedback equipment can be taken home for convenience. In one study conducted by Dr. Joseph Sargent, head of the Department of Internal Medicine at the Menninger Clinic in Topeka, not only did the biofeedback method prove successful in reducing or eliminating headache in the vast majority of women, but 75 percent of them also didn't even need to rely on the meters within a month after starting. After training themselves with the help of the instruments, they were soon able to get along without them and to raise their hand temperature, and thus the blood flow, with no outside aid. It's a little like learning to ride a bicycle. Once you learn how, the technique of keeping your balance seems reflexive, although it actually has taken a carefully learned system of signals to learn to keep from falling over.

We now have rooms in the Diamond Headache Clinic made as dark and as soundproof as possible where patients can learn biofeedback. And we've arranged for monitors to be leased to our patients until they learn to get along without them.

Since headache pain starts with abnormal constriction or narrowing of the blood vessels in the head, biofeedback helps by reversing the process. Biofeedback produces a state of relaxation that increases blood flow and causes the blood vessels in the head to "warm up" and dilate normally, instead of dilating wildly and causing a migraine.

Next, I'll show you some simple exercises that can help you relax. But remember, as with any new skill, practice is most important.

DIAPHRAGMATIC BREATHING EXERCISES

At our clinic in Chicago, we've found that learning to breath in a relaxed manner can be very helpful when used on a daily basis to prevent headaches or at least to decrease the severity of those attacks that still do occur. Originally these breathing techniques were developed as an aid to our biofeedback exercises, but many patients have found that they work well on their own as well. If you are participating in biofeedback training, they are a must.

Proper breathing promotes relaxation, which may prevent headaches by promoting stable blood-calcium levels. When people are anxious, they tend to hyperventilate, take short, rapid breaths. The result is that hormonal secretions lower their blood-calcium levels. This can cause the muscle cramping and other physiological changes that may lead to headache.

Keep in mind that relaxation is subjective and very personal, so that not all relaxation exercises will necessarily feel right to you. Try them all initially, but feel free to use only those that you like or that help you the most.

The following breathing exercises are designed to help you to achieve the relaxation response. These exercises should be done many times a day (especially when stress levels are high) to help relieve tension and pain as well as to clear the mind.

The basic technique to all our breathing exercises is diaphragmatic breathing. This is nothing more than learning to use the diaphragm at the bottom of your lungs to inhale and exhale, instead of your upper chest. The diaphragm is a partition that separates the chest and abdomen; it contains muscle and connective tissue. Diaphragmatic breathing exercises promote relaxation and can be used by anyone, with or without headaches, in order to relieve stress.

Use the abdominal muscles to enhance the movement of the diaphragm. By using the abdominal muscles we rest the muscles associated with emergency breathing—those in the upper chest, neck, and shoulders.

All breathing exercises should be done by taking slow, gentle, deep breaths. When exhaling, always contract (suck in) the abdomen (your tummy). When inhaling, always distend (push out) the abdomen, as if filling a balloon.

Exercise 1

Exhale completely, pulling in the abdominal muscles.

1. Begin a low, gentle inhalation through the nose while slowly and simultaneously distending the abdomen. Imagine that you are breathing in a sense of ease, quiet energy, and well-being. Take

this breath down to the bottom of your lungs, allowing your chest to expand slightly. Do not allow your shoulders to rise.

2. When your lungs feel full, allow a slow, smooth transition between inhaling and exhaling.

3. Begin to exhale through your mouth slowly, while contracting the abdominal muscles, again remembering not to move your shoulders. While

Diaphragmatic Breathing Exercises

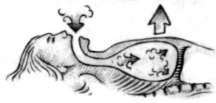

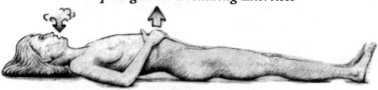

When inhaling, always distend (push out) the abdomen.

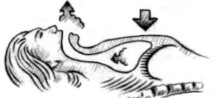

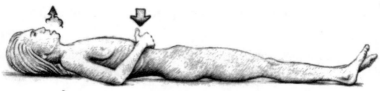

When exhaling, always contract (pull in) the abdomen.

exhaling, imagine that you are bringing up from within you any discomfort and muscle tension with your breath. Blow your breath gently away from you through your mouth, allowing a sense of quiet to take over your body.

4. Repeat the above steps two more times.

Exercise 2

Exhale completely, pulling in your abdominal muscles.

1. Inhale through your nose slowly, deeply, and diaphragmatically. Let your eyes close.

2. When your lungs feel full, allow a slow, smooth transition between inhaling and exhaling.

3. Exhale fully and completely through your nose, making sure to get the last bit of air out of your lungs by contracting your abdominal muscles.

4. Inhale through your nose again. While focusing on your inhalation, picture the number 1 in your mind.

5. Hold your breath for three seconds.

6. Exhale slowly and completely while picturing the number 2.

7. Inhale, picturing the number 3 and focusing on your inhalation.

8. Hold your breath for three seconds.

9. Exhale slowly, visualizing the number 4.

10. Continue the same process, each time using the next number until you reach the number 8.

11. Focusing on the sense of quiet inside you, slowly let your eyes open.

Exercise 3

Exhale completely, pulling in the abdominal muscles.

1. Take a slow, deep, diaphragmatic breath and, as you inhale, say the number 5 to yourself.
2. Exhale slowly, fully, and diaphragmatically.
3. Say the number 4 to yourself and inhale.
4. As you exhale, say to yourself: "I am more relaxed now than I was at number 5." Be sure not to rush the thought.
5. Say the number 3 to yourself while inhaling.
6. As you exhale, say to yourself: "I am more relaxed now than I was at number 4."
7. Continue this process until you have counted down to the number 1.

Exercise 4

Imagine that your lungs are divided horizontally into three parts.

1. Take a deep, diaphragmatic breath. Visualize the lowest part of your lungs filled with air. Use only your diaphragm; your chest and shoulders should remain still.
2. Imagine the middle part of your lungs filling with air and, as you visualize the expansion, allow your rib cage to expand.

3. Visualize the upper part of your lungs filling with air and your lungs becoming completely full. Allow your shoulders to rise slightly.

4. Slowly begin to exhale, allowing your shoulders to drop slightly. Visualize the air leaving the top portion of your lungs.

5. Visualize the air leaving the middle portion of your lungs and feel your rib cage contract.

6. Pull in your abdomen to force out the last bit of air from the bottom of your lungs.

7. Repeat the exercise three times.

PROGRESSIVE RELAXATION EXERCISE

This relaxation technique teaches you to sense when certain muscles may be subconsciously tensed. It works by allowing you to compare how a muscle feels when it is tensed deliberately with how it feels when it is relaxed.

Think of your muscles in groups (such as all the muscles in your arms, legs, or chest). Focusing on one group of muscles at a time, allow all the tension and discomfort to flow away from these muscles. In order to do this, you may use imagery, autogenic exercises, and breathing exercises in any combination. For example, you may imagine your muscles are being massaged, warmed by a heating pad, smoothed out, or just becoming heavy and loose.

To begin this exercise, find a comfortable position and take three deep but gentle breaths. As described above, focus on each of the following areas in turn and allow all tension and discomfort to flow away from them. Pay special attention to the areas in *italics*.

1. Feet
2. Lower legs
3. Upper legs, with special attention to *inner thighs*
4. *Buttocks muscles and sphincters*
5. Lower back and stomach
6. Chest
7. Upper back
8. *Shoulders*
9. *Neck*
10. *Base of skull*
11. *Jaw*
12. Tongue
13. *Temples*
14. Eyes
15. *Forehead*
16. Scalp

At the end of the exercise, take two deep, slow breaths, exhaling any tension that might remain and inhaling a sense of well-being and energy.

Now one at a time, sense all the muscle groups. Are they all in the relaxed state? If not, work on them some more.

AUTOGENIC EXERCISE

Autogenic training is a form of relaxation training that employs visualization. It was developed by the research of a German psychiatrist, Johannes Schultz.

Begin by finding a comfortable position and taking three deep but gentle breaths. Repeat the following phrases three times to yourself slowly and in a relaxed manner:

Both my arms are very heavy.

Both my legs are very heavy.

Both my hands are very heavy and warm.

Both my feet are very heavy and warm.

Breathing slow and regular.

My heartbeat is slow and regular.

My midsection is relaxed and comfortable.

My shoulders and neck are loose and comfortable.

My jaw and tongue are very relaxed and loose.

My forehead is smooth and comfortable.

My eyes and scalp are heavy and relaxed.

My mind is calm and quiet.

My entire body feels comfortable and relaxed.

I am alert in an easy, quiet, and relaxed way.

End the exercise by taking two deep, slow breaths, as if you are inhaling a sense of well-being and energy and exhaling any tension that remains. With these two deep, slow breaths, give yourself an inner smile.

IMAGERY EXERCISES

The mind is a very powerful tool in the process of relaxation. A thought can elicit a physiological response. For instance, picture a lemon. In your mind go through the process of touching it, slicing it, smelling it, then taking a taste of it. This imagery will often make you salivate, even pucker.

You can put this valuable phenomenon to use in bringing about relaxation. By simply allowing your mind to imagine some very pleasant, quiet, calming scene, you can produce the physical responses that would be present in those surroundings. The imagined place can be either a real one that you find particularly pleasant or one conjured up in your imagination. In either case you should imagine a place that gives you a sense of well-being and warmth, such as a lovely, sunny beach, a warm, inviting fireplace, or a cozy, safe room.

Before beginning the exercise, take three deep, slow and flowing breaths. Move yourself into the picture you are imagining. Try to see, hear, smell, and feel every detail of the image as though you were there. Bring your senses close to the details of the image. Experience as much of the imagery situation as possible. Get involved in the process of being there.

At the end of the exercise, take two deep, slow breaths, exhaling any tension that might be left, inhaling a sense of well-being and energy. Give yourself an inner smile.

EYE STRETCHES

These simple exercises can be done quickly and easily without significantly interrupting your activities. They should be done regularly to improve muscle tone and to help avoid strain and fatigue. It is best to do them even more often when stress is greater.

Sitting comfortably upright at a table or desk, take a deep, gentle diaphragmatic breath.

1. Close your eyes and exhale fully and completely.
2. Leaning forward, rest your elbows on the table in front of you, cupping your hands gently over your eyes with the heels of your hands resting on your cheekbones. (Do not put any pressure on your eyeballs.)

3. Remain in this position while taking three slow, deep diaphragmatic breaths.

4. Remove your hands and slowly open your eyes.

5. Without moving your head, slowly raise your eyes toward the ceiling as far as you can without straining. Slowly inhale.

6. Lower your eyes toward the floor as far as you can without straining. Slowly exhale, allowing the tension to flow out of your eyes and face.

7. Repeat Steps 5 and 6 twice.

8. Cup your eyes with your hands, close your eyes, and take three deep, gentle and complete diaphragmatic breaths.

9. Remove your hands and slowly open your eyes.

EXERCISE

Exercise is another nonmedical therapy that in some cases can help prevent menstrual headaches and alleviate general PMS symptoms. Some women have noted a decrease in the severity and frequency of their headaches and PMS symptoms if they exercised aerobically twenty to thirty minutes per day, for three to seven days during the premenstrual phase.

Researchers believe that exercise may lower levels of estrogen in the body. Interestingly enough, female athletes have been found to start menstruating later and enter menopause earlier than non-exercisers. Lower estrogen levels among female athletes is probably the reason.

Since high levels of estrogen have been linked to menstrual headaches, the estrogen-lowering effect of physical activity could explain why women suffer fewer severe headaches when they do work out.

There are simple exercises that you can do at your desk to help relieve the buildup of muscle tension and the resulting headache. Neck rolls are the most effective of these. Gently move the head in a circle. Remember, be gentle. Move slowly. Faster is not better. Now, reverse the direction of the rolls. Sixty seconds of neck rolls can make a world of difference in your muscle tension.

Shoulder rolls are great for loosening up the muscles of the upper back. Make your shoulders describe a circle together. Then, have them describe the same circle, only 180 degrees apart. Now reverse.

Transcutaneous Electrical Nerve Stimulator—TENS

Like many modern headache remedies, electrical stimulation of nerves to block pain sensations is as old as human history. Back in A.D. 46, the Roman physician Scribonius Largus described the first electrical headache remedy—a live torpedo fish. The torpedo fish is a type of sting ray that stuns or kills its prey with electrical shocks.

This is known as counter-irritation. TENS uses this technique to help block pain. The TENS device has small electrodes that are taped to the skin over the area of discomfort. The unit generates a pulsating electrical current to block the pain.

Some pain specialists have advocated the use of TENS units for nondrug treatment of headache. However, the majority of headache specialists and neurologists do not recommend this modality for the treatment of headaches because they find it minimally effective. In our experience it is of questionable and expensive help for a select group of patients.

ACUPUNCTURE

Acupuncture is based upon Chinese health maintenance and healing traditions thousands of years old. The basic idea is that all disease is the result of imbalances in the basic life force, known as Qui (pronounced "chee"). According to the theory, fine stainless steel needles placed into the top layer of the skin over any one of some 720 points on the body adjust these imbalances and can correct most of mankind's ailments. Because the needles are so fine, and they are usually placed into only the top layer of skin, the patient feels only a small, initial prick at insertion.

There are patients that may be helped by acupuncture. But as a general method, I have found acupuncture disappointing. It has only a limited amount of use in headache treatment; the results are very transient, not permanent, non-economical. Although I have used this treatment for many years, I have recently stopped using it at my own office because of the consistent lack of success.

SLEEP HABITS

Headache sufferers might be wise to avoid sleeping late on weekends and holidays, particularly if they normally drink caffeine-containing beverages like coffee or tea in the morning. Caffeine has a vasoconstrictive, or blood-vessel-narrowing effect, to which they may be accustomed. If you sleep later than usual, the caffeine deprivation can trigger headaches. At our clinic, patients are advised to get up at the same time each day. If they would like to go back to bed on weekends or holidays, they should eat or drink something such as a glass of orange juice or milk before returning to bed.

Another reason to rise and shine instead of snoozing late is that studies have shown that headaches can result from longer-than-normal sleep periods. When headaches begin during sleep, they usually do so during the REM (rapid eye movement), or the dream phase, of sleep, which occurs at regular intervals during the night. Holiday and weekend headaches may stem from the fact that more REM sleep phases occur during longer sleeping periods.

Napping can also pose a problem. While a nap may rid you of an existing headache, you don't want to nap if you're headache-free, because napping often causes migraines. Why? Because the sleep state causes blood levels of the neurotransmitter hormone serotonin to rise, and rising serotonin levels are a major cause of migraines.

Once you are caught in the middle of a migraine attack, however, sleep may be a great remedy. It may even reduce your need for migraine medication. In fact, a preliminary study presented at the International Headache Congress in 1991 showed that people with mild migraines with no accompanying nausea or vomiting found relief in a nap. These patients were able to eliminate or at least delay the need for normal migraine medicine when they napped.

But how do you fall asleep when your head is pounding? Find a quiet, dark place and lie down. If you can't fall asleep easily, try counting backward from 100. Or visualize lying on a warm beach with the surf gently lapping at your feet.

If you really can't fall asleep, don't worry. In many cases simply lying down and resting will work just as well.

Whenever you do sleep, sleep straight. Sleeping in an awkward position or even on your stomach can cause the muscles in your neck to contract and trigger a headache. Sleeping on your back is your best bet.

AVOIDING HEADACHE TRIGGERS

Although migraine has a definite organic basis, psychological factors do play a crucial role as a trigger of individual attacks. There is substantial evidence that points to prolonged stress as a contributor to the frequency of migraine attacks. When I interview a patient for the first time, I ask questions about the job, school, marriage, and   relationships with parents, children, in-laws, and friends. By establishing a rapport early with the patient, I allow her to open up to me regarding any personal problems that may contribute to her headaches.

In taking a patient's history, many times I ask questions about when their headaches first developed. Some patients will relay that their headaches started after a long period of emotional conflict, a perceived loss, bereavement, physical illness, or disruption of their social support systems, including divorce, loss of job, etc. The patient may require counseling in order to help cope with these different emotional events.

You must realize and identify stressful triggers; try not to take on too many chores or challenges as this will only add to your migraine problem. Learning to identify the triggers and cope with stress is very important in the total treatment regimen in the headache patient.

Foods: From 25 to 45 percent of my patients tell me their attacks are precipitated by eating certain foods. At the Diamond Headache Clinic we use a selective diet (see appendix I). At least 40 percent of my patients have found this diet effective in reducing the frequency, severity, and duration of their acute headaches.

Whether certain foodstuffs can precipitate migraine is controversial. The results of an elimination diet have been reported as positive by some and negative by others in my own studies (as well as in studies by other experts). Some patients will comment that at one time a food will cause a reaction while at another time the same food will not cause a headache. A trigger factor may only have the potential to cause a headache if combined with another trigger factor. For example, a woman may not get a headache when ingesting tyramine-containing foods except when she is experiencing hormonal fluctuations, such as those that occur during menstruation.

The mechanism by which diet provokes headaches is obscure but probably not an allergic phenomenon. Many of the foods commonly cited as triggering migraine attacks contain what we call vasoactive amines. Vasoactive amines earned their name because they influence the blood vessels. These amines, or monoamines, are constantly identified as migraine triggers; even small amounts of these chemicals can cause an attack in someone who is susceptible.

Chocolate is considered by most headache experts to be a major cause of migraine attacks. These attacks may take as long as twenty-four hours to develop. The vasoactive substance in chocolate is phenylethylamine.

Between 40 and 60 percent of migraine patients believe that the consumption of alcoholic beverages is a definite cause of their migraines. When patients have noted their diet triggers, alcohol is probably the most common factor reported. It is believed that the alcohol itself may not be a factor, but the impurities in major alcohol beverages cause the problem. Wines, vodka, light scotches, and whiskeys have a lower impurity or congener content and therefore can be tolerated by some migraine patients when ingested in small amounts. I should reiterate that I am not talking about hangover headaches.

Tyramine is the most frequently implicated vasoactive amine in migraine attacks. It has been thought that tyramine also triggers headaches by causing the release of chemicals known as catecholamines, one of which is epinephrine. Epinephrine is present in the nerve endings as well as the adrenal gland. The release of the catecholamines is responsible for, and has been shown to provoke, both an increase in blood pressure and migraine attacks in certain individuals.

The foods that do contain high concentrations of tyramine are matured and ripened cheeses, such as Camembert, Brie, cheddar, Parmesan, Roquefort, bleu brick, Stilton, and the blue-veined cheeses such as Danish blue, blue Stilton, and cheddar. Processed cheeses (cream cheese, American cheese, cottage cheese) have lower concentrations of tyramine. Yogurt and sour cream all have light levels unless these products have been allowed to ferment for extended periods of time. Dried, salted herring and other salted fish contain large amounts of tyramine, as do cured meats such as bologna, salami, and certain sausages. Brewer's yeast also contains a fair amount of tyramine and is present in beers, Chianti, and several smoked meat products. Foods that have been inadequately refrigerated will cause an increase in the amounts of tyramine.

It's important for patients with headaches to do their own testing with a low-tyramine diet. Some patients may be more sensitive to chocolate and cheese than others, and other patients may note that they do not get headaches after eating such foods as pizza. If you know that one food definitely causes a headache then try to avoid it.

MSG: Monosodium glutamate, MSG, is used extensively as a flavor enhancer and as a food additive in Chinese cuisine. It is present in large amounts in canned, frozen, diet, and prepared foods such as snacks and fast food. Soy sauce also contains a substantial amount. MSG is frequently difficult to identify in some foods because of the variety of terms used by the manufacturer. These terms include hydrolyzed vegetable protein, calcium caseinate, hydrolyzed plant protein, protein hydrolyzate, natural flavor, and glutavene kombu extract. When present in high amounts, MSG induces adverse reactions in about one-third of normal individuals. This is described as the Chinese Restaurant Syndrome, and symptoms include dizziness, diarrhea, nausea, abdominal cramps, paraesthesia, a pins-and-needles sensation of the mouth and palate, pressure pain in the neck and shoulders, and severe headache. These symptoms develop within twenty minutes of ingestion. A large number of migraine patients are susceptible to MSG headaches and develop a throbbing or unilateral headache within fifteen to thirty minutes after eating a food flavored with small amounts of MSG. Many migraine sufferers cannot distinguish attacks of MSG-related migraine from their typical migraine attacks.

Nitrites (Hot Dog Headache): Nitrites are preservatives found in processed and cured meats such as frankfurters, ham, bologna, bacon, salami, and in smoked fish, such as lox. Sodium nitrite is used as a food coloring and preservative. A number of individuals develop headaches minutes to hours after eating foods containing nitrites. Some people have described this as the Hot Dog Headache. The headache usually affects both sides and the front of the head and is usually throbbing in nature. Facial flushing may also occur. Many migraineurs may experience nitrite-provoked headaches.

Caffeine: Very few patients indicate that their migraine headaches are produced by consumption of caffeine-containing products. In fact, when combined with different analgesics or ergotamines, caffeine will usually help abort an acute migraine. Some patients rely on heavy doses of a caffeine-containing analgesic, only to find that when they discontinue use they suffer from caffeine withdrawal. Physical symptoms of withdrawal tend to develop in people who ingest large amounts of caffeine in coffee, teas, colas, or in medications containing caffeine. The most frequently reported symptoms of caffeine withdrawal include headache, drowsiness, fatigue, anxiety, irritability, restlessness, difficulty concentrating, clouded thinking, and nausea.

These symptoms are promptly relieved by the ingestion of more caffeine. Caffeine-withdrawal headaches usually occur within eight to sixteen hours following cessation of caffeine. Such headaches can usually peak at twenty-four to forty-eight hours, but may last several days to a week. Individuals who ingest substantial quantities of caffeine during the work week may develop withdrawal headaches on the weekend. For many migraine patients, caffeine deprivation may be responsible for the headaches they experience upon awakening.

Aspartame: Headache is probably the most prevalent consumer complaint related to aspartame (such as Nutrasweet). About 8 percent of headache patients link aspartame to headache pain. Clinical trials have been controversial as to its effects. If you are sensitive to aspartame or any products containing it, you should omit its use.

Cold Foods (Ice Cream Headache): A severe, brief, frontal headache can occur after eating ice cream. It can actually happen when any cold substance is applied to the roof of the mouth. The pain is usually dull and throbbing. It can be felt in the face, throat, or head and often radiates all over the head, since the fifth cranial nerve carries the sensation from the front of the mouth and distributes it along its many branches. The pain lasts for only a few minutes. This kind of head pain may be helped by slowly cooling the mouth with small amounts of the cold substance. People who suffer from migraine and cluster headaches are especially prone to the ice cream headache.

Hunger and Hypoglycemia: Changes in blood sugar may precipitate an acute migraine attack. However, it is not necessary for you to follow a strict hypoglycemic diet, as it will only offer sporadic help. But if you do suffer from migraines or other chronic headaches, you must realize that it is vital for you to maintain regularity in your daily living patterns to avoid headaches. You should eat three well-balanced meals daily at set times and avoid oversleeping. It is important for you to avoid the tendency to sleep later on Saturday or Sunday morning. Waking up late can cause you to skip breakfast, which will lower your body's normal blood sugar level and may trigger a headache.

Exercise (Effort Headache): Other headache triggers include fatigue and exertion. Fatigue caused by exertion or lack of adequate rest can induce a migraine headache. Effort migraine, as it is known, is described as bilateral throbbing with typical migraine features; it can develop in some people when they exercise, particularly if the exercise is excessive or violent. Activities such as running, playing football, weightlifting, or dancing can precipitate some attacks. These attacks will occur almost immediately after the activity. Tension-type headaches may also be induced by exercise and of course those involved in contact sports have the potential for posttraumatic headache. For patients experiencing an acute headache, even the mildest form of exercise can exacerbate the degree of pain, usually due to the increased blood flow to the already dilated arteries. Prolonged exercise may produce an intense headache with nausea and vomiting, which could be related to dehydration or temporary hypoglycemia.

Headaches due to exercise are usually vascular in nature. Exercise induced headache is described as very severe but of short duration lasting from a few seconds to a few minutes. One form of avoiding an exercise-induced migraine is to perform a five- to ten-minute warmup before the exercise and include a brief cool-down period after the main exercise period. Headache patients should start conditioning gradually, because pushing above one's normal fitness level can precipitate a headache. It is wise to avoid exercising in the middle of the day when the sunlight and heat may add to the potential for getting a headache.

Visual Stimuli: Many patients will comment about headache being triggered by extremes of bright light and loud noises. Even the nuances of light in a television or movie screen can aggravate a headache. If bright light causes headache, try buying sunglasses with an ultraviolet coating; prescription eyeglasses may also be ordered with this protective coating.

Odors: Many female migraine patients will complain of odor sensitivity during a migraine attack, particularly during aura. They will also state that particular odors, including cigar or cigarette smoke, paint, gasoline fumes, tar, or asphalt may trigger an attack. Unfortunately it may be the pleasant odor from a perfume, cologne, aftershave lotion, or fragrances added to hair spray and shampoo that can trigger a headache. Friends and families of migraine sufferers should be particularly sensitive to any problems their loved one experiences with specific odors.

Smoking: For about one-third of my patients, smoking initiates or exacerbates the symptoms of headache. Chronic daily headaches are more common among patients who smoke than nonsmokers. There also appears to be a high incidence of smokers in groups of cluster-headache patients. I advise all of my patients who smoke to stop smoking for obvious health reasons and I always instruct my cluster patients to avoid smoking during a cluster period.

Medications: Some medication used for coexisting medical illnesses may trigger a headache, including reserpine, nitrates, and other vasodilators (used in cardiac medications), indomethacin, and hormone supplements. I have also seen many migraine attacks precipitated by the use of illicit drugs, especially cocaine or heroin.

Seasonal Factors: Many patients identify seasonal and weather changes as headache triggers. There is a marked tendency for cluster headaches during spring and fall, and many migraine sufferers note that adverse weather conditions will influence an acute attack. There has also been a correlation between headaches and hot, dry winds. However, we do not recommend that patients buy expensive machines or move to other areas; these solutions may only lead to other triggers.

Other: Many patients will complain of severe head pain when they take a plane or stay in regions of high altitude, such as on a ski vacation. Motion sickness has also been known to precipitate migraine, especially in children. Up to 60 percent of migraine patients report a history of motion sickness as children. In either case, consult your doctor before planning your next trip.

$\mathcal{A}$ PPENDIX I

THE DIAMOND HEADACHE CLINIC'S DIETARY PLAN FOR HEADACHE PATIENTS

Many headache sufferers have been helped enormously by restricting tyramine and other vasoactive substances from their daily diets. Most people will find that relatively minor adjustments in their eating habits will be sufficient.

The following table lists food to avoid or limit, with plausible substitutions where applicable. Of course, as with any diet, you should check with your physician first and be sure not to neglect any other dietary restrictions or mandates that you may require.

LOW-TYRAMINE HEADACHE DIET

What Is Tyramine?

Tyramine is produced in food from the natural breakdown of the amino acid tyrosine. Tyramine is never added to foods. Tyramine levels increase in foods when they are aged, fermented, stored for long periods of time, or not fresh. All food, especially high-protein foods, should be prepared and eaten fresh. Do not eat leftovers held for more than one day.

Each day eat three meals with a snack at night or six small meals spread throughout the day.

MSG and nitrates do not have the same effect as tyramine-containing foods but can cause headache in many people. The foods listed in the Use with Caution column have smaller amounts of tyramine or other vasoactive compounds. You need to avoid these foods if you are taking an MAO inhibitor (Marplan, Nardil, Parnate).

Caffeinated beverages may be used only in allowed amounts.

Each person may have different sensitivities to a certain level of tyramine or other vasoactive compounds in foods. If you are not on an MAO inhibitor you should test the restricted-use foods in limited amounts.

Foods	Allowed	Use with Caution	Avoid
Beverages	Decaffeinated coffee, fruit juices, club soda, caffeine-free carbonated beverages.	Limit caffeinated beverages to no more than 2 servings per day: coffee and tea: 1 cup = 1 serving carbonated beverages and chocolate milk or hot cocoa: 12 oz. = 1 serving. Limit alcoholic beverages to one serving: 4 oz. Riesling Wine, 1.5 oz. vodka or scotch per day = 1 serving per day.	Alcoholic beverages: Chianti, sherry, burgundy, vermouth, beer, ale, and nonalcoholic fermented beverages. All others not specified in caution column.

Meat, Fish, Poultry, Eggs	Freshly purchased and prepared meats, fish, and poultry.	Bacon, sausage, hot dogs, corned beef, bologna, ham, any luncheon meats with nitrites.	Aged, dried, fermented, salted, smoked, or pickled products. Pepperoni, salami, and liverwurst.
	Eggs.	Meats with tenderizer added.	
	Tuna fish, tuna salad (with allowed ingredients).	Caviar.	Nonfresh meat or liver.
			Pickled herring.
Dairy	Milk: Whole, 2%, or skim.	Parmesan or Romano as a garnish (2 tsp.) or minor ingredient.	Aged cheese: Blue, brick, brie, cheddar, Swiss, Roquefort, Stilton, mozzarella, provolone, and emmentaler.
	Cheese: American, cottage, farmer, ricotta, cream cheese, Velveeta, low-fat processed cheese.	Yogurt, buttermilk, sour cream: 1/2 cup per day.	
Breads, Cereals, Pasta	Commercially prepared yeast products.	Homemade yeast-leavened breads and coffee cake.	Any with restricted ingredients.
	Products leavened with baking powder: biscuits, pancakes, coffee cakes, etc.	Sourdough breads.	
	All hot and dry cereals.		
	All pasta: spaghetti, rotini, ravioli (with allowed ingredients), macaroni, and egg noodles.		

Foods	Allowed	Use with Caution	Avoid
Vegetables	Asparagus, string beans, beets, carrots, spinach, pumpkin, tomatoes, squash, zucchini, broccoli, potatoes, onions cooked in food, snow peas, navy beans, soy beans, any not on list to restrict.	Raw onion.	Fava or broad beans, sauerkraut, fermented soy products like miso tofu, and pickles. Soy sauce.
Fruits	Apple, applesauce, cherries, apricots, peaches, any not on restricted list.	Limit intake to 1/2 cup per day from each group: Citrus: orange, grapefruit, tangerine, pineapple, lemon, and lime. Avocados, banana, figs, raisins, papaya, passion fruit, and red plums.	
Nuts and Seeds			All nuts: Peanuts, peanut butter, pumpkin seeds, sesame seeds, walnuts, pecans, etc.
Soups	Soups made from allowed ingredients, homemade broths.	Canned soups with autolyzed or hydrolyzed yeast, meat extracts, or monosodium glutamate (MSG).	
Desserts and Sweets	Any made with allowed foods and ingredients: sugar, jelly, jam, honey, hard candies, cakes, cookies.	Chocolate based products: Ice cream (1 cup), pudding (1 cup), cookies (1 cup), cakes (3" cube), and chocolate candies (1/2 oz.).	Mincemeat pie.
Ingredients	Any not listed.		

Can I Eat Vegetarian on the Low-Tyramine Headache Diet?

In most cases the answer is yes. Many people are concerned that the restriction of cheese, nuts, and seed may make it hard to get enough protein.

First you need to define what kind of vegetarian you are:

	Foods Excluded	*Foods Included*
Lacto-ovo-vegetarian	milk, milk products like yogurt and cheese* (lacto), eggs (ovo), fruits, grains, legumes (soy beans, garbanzo beans, lentils, chickpeas), nuts*, and seeds*	beef, poultry, fish
Vegan	fruits, grains, legumes, nuts*, and seeds*	beef, poultry, fish, milk and milk products, eggs

* Restricted on the low-tyramine diet. Refer to the low-tyramine diet guidelines for more details.

If you eat small amounts of animal products like fish and poultry and include legumes and grains, you are very likely to have an adequate protein intake.

For lacto-ovo vegetarians, dairy products (allowed on the low-tyramine diet) and eggs provide complete proteins. Including these foods with grains and legumes will provide adequate amounts of protein for most people.

For vegans, the combined proteins from legumes and grains will provide complete proteins. These food groups do not have to be eaten in precise amounts or at the same meal to provide complete proteins for the day.

Overall, the foods allowed on the low-tyramine diet will provide most every type of vegetarian with a nutritious diet.

$\mathcal{A}$ PPENDIX II

THE HEADACHE CALENDAR

One of the most invaluable tools in preventing headaches is identifying the triggers of acute attacks. All Diamond Headache Clinic patients are asked to maintain a daily diary in which they list the presence or absence of a headache, the time of onset, and the degree of severity. Also, they are asked to note any specific factors that could have contributed to the headache, including food items, emotional aspects, menses, and weather. Finally, the patients are asked to record the medications used to relieve the headache, the amount of medication consumed, and the degree of relief that was obtained. A sample of the headache calendar follows.

HEADACHE CALENDAR

PATIENT'S NAME:

DIAMOND HEADACHE CLINIC, LTD.

Date	Time Onset Ending (insert hr. and A.M./P.M.)	(*1) Severity of Headache	(*2) Psychic and Physical Factors	(*3) Food and Drink Excesses	Medication Taken and Dosage	(*4) Relief of Headache

HEADACHE KEYS

(*1) SEVERITY SCALE

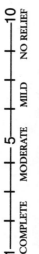

1	5	10
NONE	MILD	MODERATE	SEVERE

(*2) PSYCHIC & PHYSICAL FACTORS

1 - Emotional Upset/Family or Friends
2 - Emotional Upset/Occupation
3 - Business/Reversal
4 - Business/Success
5 - Vacation Days
6 - Weekends
7 - Strenuous Exercise
8 - Strenuous Labor
9 - High Altitude Location
10 - Anticipation Anxiety
11 - Crisis/Serious
12 - Post-Crisis Period
13 - New Job/Position
14 - New Move
15 - Menstrual Days
16 - Physical Illness
17 - Oversleeping
18 - Weather
19 - Fasting
20 - Missing a Meal
21 - Other

(*4) RELIEF SCALE

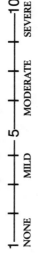

1	5	10
COMPLETE	MODERATE	MILD	NO RELIEF

(*3) FOOD & DRINK EXCESSES

A - Ripened Cheeses (Pizza)
B - Herring
C - Chocolate
D - Vinegar
E - Fermented Foods (pickled or marinated)
       (sour cream/yogurt)
F - Freshly Baked Yeast Products
G - Nuts (Peanut Butter)
H - Monosodium Glutamate (Chinese Foods)
I - Pods of Broad Beans
J - Onions
K - Canned Figs
L - Citrus Foods
M - Bananas
N - Pork
O - Caffeinated Beverages (Cola)
P - Avocado
Q - Fermented Sausage (Cured Cold Cuts)
R - Chicken Livers
S - Wine
T - Alcohol
U - Beer

GLOSSARY

ABDOMINAL MIGRAINE—A type of migraine in which the pain is not located in the head but rather in the upper part of the abdomen. The pain lasts only a few hours. Those afflicted with abdominal migraine are usually children, mostly girls with a family history of migraine. Like migraine headaches, the attacks of abdominal migraine are recurrent and are often accompanied by a headache.

ACUPUNCTURE—Acupuncture is an ancient Chinese remedy for a variety of illnesses. It is based on the theory that by stimulating nerves one can block pain. The puncture acts as a counterirritant to stop the painful impulses from radiating up the spinal cord. Some patients have responded to the use of acupuncture in headache treatment, but the overall results have been insignificant.

ALPHA AGONISTS—These drugs, which have shown some effectiveness in migraine, were originally used in the treatment of hypertension. The most commonly used alpha agonist, clonidine, has shown marginal success in migraine therapy, except for those patients with a particular sensitivity to tyramine-containing foods.

ANEURYSM—An aneurysm is a weakness in the wall of a blood vessel, which at some critical point may balloon out and rupture. Unless the aneurysm is large, patients will rarely exhibit symptoms unless it ruptures. It is essential to take a complete history of a patient with a sudden onset of headache, as it may mean aneurysm. The symptoms of chronic headaches, including migraine, however, do not resemble the symptoms of a ruptured aneurysm.

ANTIDEPRESSANTS—As their name suggests, these medications are used for depression. For patients with chronic headache, these drugs are useful for their mood-elevating properties as well as their analgesic actions. The drugs are especially helpful for those headache patients with a sleep disturbance.

ANXIETY HEADACHE—This is a form of chronic tension-type headache which is related to an underlying anxiety. The anxiety may be indicated by job complaints or stress. The patient may complain of a sleep disturbance in the form of difficulty falling asleep.

AURA—The aura of migraine consists of neurological signs of an impending headache. Usually the aura refers to a variety of visual symptoms, including seeing bright or flashing lights, zigzag lines, distorted size, shape, and location, and even losing part of the visual field. Patients may also experience hallucinations in hearing and smell prior to the onset of the migraine attack. Other patients may notice numbness or tingling in their arms or legs before the migraine headache starts.

BASILAR ARTERY MIGRAINE—Occurring commonly in young women, basilar-artery migraine is often misdiagnosed due to the associated confusion, unsteady gait, and dizziness. The examining physician may think the patient is mentally disturbed, drunk, or drug intoxicated. This type of migraine affects the circulation of blood to parts of the brain supplied by the basilar artery. The headache usually affects the back of the head, and the patient will complain of nausea, double-vision, and slurred speech, as well as the symptoms previously mentioned. During an acute attack, some patients may lose consciousness. Many patients may show a family history for similar headaches.

BETA BLOCKERS—These drugs act by blocking the action of certain substances, such as adrenaline, found in the body. Previously used in the treatment of hypertension and cardiac problems, these drugs have demonstrated their effectiveness in preventing migraine. The only beta blockers approved for migraine treatment are propranolol and timolol. Patients with respiratory problems may not be able to tolerate those beta blockers, which are not selective, and should be started on a cardioselective beta blocker, such as metoprolol.

BIOFEEDBACK—Biofeedback is a technique that trains the patient to control a previously unused or involuntarily controlled function of the body, such as heart rate, blood pressure, muscle tension, and temperature. It is used in a variety of medical conditions and is particularly effective with migraine and tension headaches. The control is achieved through training with a monitor that measures these bodily functions. The monitor feeds back information about the bodily function to the patient, and through various methods (diaphragmatic breathing, relaxation phases) the patient learns to control that particular function. Biofeedback also uses self-hypnotic techniques or progressive relaxation.

CAFFEINE—Caffeine is commonly known as an ingredient in coffee, tea, and cola beverages. It is also a frequent ingredient in over-the-counter analgesics. In some preparations of ergotamine, caffeine is added to potentiate the absorption of the ergotamine. Unfortunately many patients overconsume caffeine, whether in beverages or over-the-counter analgesics. When the source of caffeine is skipped, the patient will experience a caffeine-withdrawal headache. These headaches most often occur when someone is fasting or on weekends when the person delays or skips a morning cup of coffee.

CALCIUM CHANNEL BLOCKERS—Calcium channel blockers are used for heart disease and for patients recovering from stroke. These drugs act by stabilizing the cranial blood vessels. By maintaining a balance in these blood vessels, they also prevent the brain from being exposed to an oxygen deficiency. Expansion of the blood vessels is acknowledged as a factor in migraine.

In migraine the most frequently used calcium channel blockers are verapamil and nimodipine. Nifedipine and diltiazem have not been particularly beneficial for migraine patients.

CLASSIC MIGRAINE—See Migraine with Aura.

CLUSTER HEADACHE—Type of vascular headache that occurs in a series or group of headaches. Cluster headaches occur more often in males. The headaches are characterized by their one-sided location, usually around one eye, and very brief duration, from a few minutes to one or two hours. The patient may experience several headaches per day for a period of one to several months.

COEXISTING MIGRAINE AND TENSION-TYPE HEADACHE—These headaches were previously classified as mixed headaches. These patients will report a history of two or more types of headaches occurring concurrently. Frequently the patients will note a daily mild type of headache, similar to a tension-type headache, and a more severe headache, occurring several times in a week or a month, which resembles migraine. Patients with these headaches are prone to habituation problems due to the frequency of their headaches. Often, they are also experiencing a concomitant depression.

COMMON MIGRAINE—See Migraine without Aura.

COMPLICATED MIGRAINE—This term refers to those migraine attacks accompanied by neurological symptoms, such as weakness or loss of feeling in the arms and legs. Some patients also will note problems with their vision. These neurological symptoms may persist longer than the actual headache. Although rare, permanent damage to the brain or retina may occur.

CONCUBINE SYNDROME—This syndrome occurs when the spouse or partner of a headache sufferer becomes caregiver and positively reinforces "pain behavior." The patient is discouraged from getting help for the headache problem so that they continue to rely on the "well" partner. This dependency role can also occur in children with headaches; in this case the caregiver is the parent, who reinforces pain behavior.

CT SCAN—Computerized axial tomography (CT scan) uses a computer that merges many X-rays from several angles into a single picture. The CT scan may be performed with or without a contrasting dye. The dye may be used to help identify a brain tumor or blood clot within the brain. CT scans are used frequently for headache patients to rule out an organic basis for their headaches.

DEPRESSION HEADACHES—These headaches are the most commonly occurring form of chronic tension-type headaches. In addition to daily or almost daily headaches, the patient will complain of a sleep disturbance in the form of frequent or early awakening. Often the patient does not outwardly appear to be depressed. Due to the frequency of the headaches, the patient may be prone to habituation problems with analgesics and barbiturates. The treatment of choice for these headaches are antidepressants, which are effective for their antidepressant action and possible analgesic effects.

ENDORPHIN/ENKEPHALIN—These substances are the body's natural pain killers. They are found throughout the body, and their discovery has opened the door to many new ways of relieving pain.

ERGOTAMINE—The ergotamine drugs are used to abort acute headaches. These drugs act on the blood vessels, preventing them from swelling. Ergotamine is available through prescription only and for administration in oral tablets, tablets for placement under the tongue, and as rectal suppositories. In order to avoid ergotamine rebound headaches, these drugs are never to be used on a daily basis.

ESTROGEN—Sex hormone produced in the ovary, placenta, testes, and possibly the adrenal glands. Estrogen is essential to the growth of the female sexual organs and also stimulates the secondary female characteristics, such as the development of full breasts and rounded hips. Estrogen levels vary within the menstrual cycle, rising dramatically from days nine to fourteen, about the time of ovulation, and then dropping dramatically from days twenty-four to twenty-eight, when menstrual flow begins. This decrease in estrogen levels is the impetus for the onset of menstrual migraine.

EXERTIONAL HEADACHE—This term refers to those headaches precipitated by some form of exertion, such as lifting, running, bending over, or straining. Exercise requires increased circulation to the muscles of the head, neck, and scalp, and may cause head pain. Most cases of exertional headaches have benign causes and can be treated effectively with indomethacin. Some exertional headaches may be a sign of organic disease, and the patient should be thoroughly examined to rule out a serious cause for the headache.

FSH—The follicle stimulating hormone (FSH) is produced by the pituitary gland. During each menstrual cycle the hormone causes an unfertilized egg in the ovary to mature in a tiny sac, the follicle. FSH levels peak about the seventh day of the menstrual cycle.

HORMONE—Hormones are the body's chemical messengers. They are produced by glands and are carried by the bloodstream to organs and tissues where they help regulate body systems such as growth, sexual development, metabolism, and the nervous system.

HOT DOG HEADACHE—Hot dogs and smoked meats such as salami contain sodium nitrite. This additive is used to preserve the color of the meat and to prevent botulism. Nitrites cause blood vessels to swell, and patients with migraine headache are especially sensitive to foods containing these substances. The headache will usually appear within forty-five minutes after ingesting the food item.

HYPERTENSION—Hypertension, or high blood pressure, is not a frequent cause of headache, unless the blood pressure is severely high.

ICE CREAM HEADACHE—This type of headache will occur when a cold substance is positioned against the back part of the roof of the mouth. It can result from ice cream or any other cold substance. The pain is very brief, lasting only a few minutes, and will be noted over the throat, head, or face. It can be very excruciating. Migraine patients may be more prone to this occurrence.

LUTEINIZING HORMONE—About the ninth day of the menstrual cycle the pituitary gland starts producing the luteinizing hormone (LH). LH causes the sac surrounding the mature egg to burst—usually around the fourteenth day of the cycle. LH levels decrease dramatically from days sixteen to eighteen.

LUTEOTROPIN—As the levels of luteinizing hormone decrease, the pituitary glands start to produce luteotropin (LTH). This hormone stimulates the ovaries to produce progesterone. The peak levels of LTH occur between days eighteen to twenty-four and dramatically decrease days twenty-six to twenty-eight.

MENOPAUSE—The strictest definition of menopause is the final termination of the menstrual cycle. However, this stage in a woman's life may last for several years, as her menses changes and finally ends. Menopausal women may also experience a variety of symptoms, including hot flashes and fatigue.

MENSTRUAL MIGRAINE—This term refers to those migraine attacks associated with the menstrual cycle. Approximately 70 percent of female migraine sufferers will relate their headaches to their menses. Menstrual migraines are linked to changing levels of estrogen and progesterone. Headaches can occur immediately before menses, during the menstrual flow, or immediately after menses. Some patients may experience a migraine at the time of ovulation. The treatment of choice for menstrual migraine are the NSAIDs, starting two days before menses and continuing throughout the flow.

MIGRAINE—Migraine is defined as a recurring headache that occurs one or more times per month and can last four to seventy-two hours. Typically migraine is a one-sided headache, described as pounding or throbbing, and of moderate to incapacitating severity. Migraine is often termed a "sick" headache since it's associated with nausea, vomiting, and sensitivity to light. Some patients experience migraine with aura, with defined warning symptoms before the actual migraine snack (see AURA). The majority of patients with migraine do not experience the aura but may note a vague premonition of an impending migraine attack.

MIGRAINE EQUIVALENTS—A migraine equivalent is a form of migraine that does not affect the head. Abdominal migraine is a typical migraine equivalent, where the pain is located in another part of the body. For a diagnosis of this condition, the patient will usually have a personal or family history of migraine. Like migraine the pain may last for a few hours and is recurrent. Medications used to treat migraine often relieve the symptoms of a migraine equivalent.

MIGRAINE WITH AURA (Classic Migraine)—Patients diagnosed with migraine with aura will have a history of an acute headache preceded by a neurological symptom, such as a visual disturbance (see AURA). The aura does not necessarily precede every migraine attack. Some elderly patients will note that the headaches have disappeared, but they are still troubled with symptoms of the aura.

MIGRAINE WITHOUT AURA (Common Migraine)— Patients with migraine without aura have never experienced the neurological warning signs of an aura. However, they may be able to predict an imminent headache by vague premonitory signs such as fatigue or burst of energy, increased or decreased appetite, or anxiety.

MONOAMINE OXIDASE INHIBITORS (MAOIs)—The MAOIs are a form of antidepressants used as a second line of action in headaches related to depression. These drugs have also been shown effective in migraine treatment. Because these drugs are known to have severe interactions with foods containing tyramine and other vasoactive substances, patients on MAOIs must adhere to a tyramine-free diet. The MAOIs also interact with other medications, such as certain narcotics, over-the-counter cold remedies, and local anesthetics used in dental surgery. Patients must be carefully instructed regarding the precautions with the MAOIs.

MRI—Magnetic resonance imaging (MRI) is a technique that has revolutionized the evaluation of headache patients. By using a strong magnet, the physician is able to obtain thousands of views of the brain, and a computer blends these pictures to produce an astounding image of the brain. Unlike a CT scan, MRI can differentiate between normal and pathological tissues, and measure the density of the tissues. MRI can also detect problems at an early stage of the disease. Another advantage of MRI is that it can be performed without injecting a dye into the body and gives a clearer picture without the risks of CT scanning.

MSG—Monosodium glutamate (MSG) is used as a flavor enhancer in some foods, including processed meat, meat tenderizers, and Chinese cuisine. MSG can cause headaches and other symptoms in susceptible people within thirty minutes of ingesting the food item. Symptoms, besides headache, include sweating, chest tightness, and pressure over the face and chest. Migraine patients may be especially sensitive to foods containing MSG.

NICOTINE—Nicotine is an essential substance in tobacco products, such as cigars and cigarettes. Because nicotine affects the blood vessels, smoking can contribute to the frequency and duration of migraine attacks. Patients with cluster headaches may often have to refrain from smoking during a series of headaches.

NONSTEROIDAL ANTI-INFLAMMATORY AGENTS (NSAIDs)—These are a group of ever-expanding drugs that are known to be effective in a variety of chronic pain problems, including headaches. Aspirin is the original NSAID. It is believed that during a headache a sterile inflammation occurs, and the headache will continue until the inflammation is resolved. The NSAIDs reduce this inflammation. The NSAIDs are the drugs of choice in the treatment of menstrual migraine. Examples of NSAIDs are ibuprofen, naproxen, naproxen sodium, fenoprofen calcium, and a host of others.

ORAL CONTRACEPTIVES—These drugs are used to prevent ovulation and therefore pregnancy. Birth control pills may contain estrogen or a combination of estrogen and progesterone. Oral contraceptives are known to increase the frequency, duration, severity, and complications of migraine.

ORGANIC HEADACHE—These headaches have a physical source for the pain, such as a brain tumor, blood clot, or infection. Traction and inflammatory headaches are also terms that describe these headaches. Some organic headaches may have serious consequences, and early diagnosis and treatment are essential. Fortunately, only 8 percent of all headaches are due to an organic cause.

ORGASMIC HEADACHE—This headache occurs at the moment of climax or orgasm in a sexual act. Most orgasmic headaches are benign and treated easily with the anti-inflammatory drugs (NSAIDs). However, they may also be due to a serious condition such as hypertension, brain hemorrhage, or tumor. Because of this it is essential that a patient experiencing a headache at orgasm urgently consult a physician for diagnosis and treatment.

OVULATION—The time during the menstrual cycle when the mature egg is released from its sac, usually around the fourteenth day. If the egg is not fertilized, the levels of estrogen and progesterone will drop about the twenty-fifth day and the lining of the uterus sloughs or falls off, resulting in the start of the menstrual flow at day twenty-eight.

PLATELET—An irregularly shaped cell that is produced in bone marrow and found in the blood where it helps in clotting. During the migraine process the platelets clump together and then stick to the walls of the blood vessels. This action causes the blood vessels to expand, leading the way to a migraine attack. Platelets are the primary source of serotonin.

PLATELET ANTAGONISTS—The platelet antagonists are agents that prevent the platelets from clumping together and sticking to the walls of the capillaries. This group of drugs has been used in migraine prevention with mixed results. The platelet antagonists sulfinpyrazone and dipridamole are most commonly used for elderly patients with headaches because they have fewer side effects.

PMS—Premenstrual syndrome (PMS) describes a group of symptoms that appears in the days or weeks preceding the onset of menstrual flow. These symptoms include headache, fatigue, acne, joint pain, weight gain, irritability, panic attacks, difficulty concentrating, sensitivity to rejection, decreased sexual desire, and paranoia.

POST PUNCTURE HEADACHE—This headache results from a variety of procedures involving a small puncture site in the spine. This procedure is used in spinal anesthesia—often during labor—and spinal taps. The headache may follow the procedure within hours or days. The probable cause of these headaches is the leakage of spinal fluid through the puncture site, causing a low-spinal-fluid pressure headache.

PREGNANCY AND HEADACHE—Migraine patients will often report that their headaches diminished or disappeared during pregnancy because of the stabilization of the hormones. Unfortunately the headaches usually will reappear after the delivery.

PROGESTERONE—Progesterone is the female hormone that helps prepare the lining of the uterus to receive and nurture a fertilized egg. It is produced by the ovaries, and with estrogen, causes the cells of the lining of the uterus to change shape and expand. The levels of progesterone increase on day fourteen of the menstrual cycle and decrease dramatically days twenty-six to twenty-eight.

PROLACTIN—Prolactin is a hormone produced by the pituitary gland. An increase in prolactin levels can cause an increase in breast size and a discharge from the nipples. An increase in the level of prolactin may be a sign of a tumor of the pituitary gland. These tumors are most often seen in young adults and can be treated effectively with medication.

PROSTAGLANDIN—The prostaglandins are fatty acids found throughout the body, which effect enlarging and narrowing of the blood vessels, stimulation of various muscles, and uterine stimulation (contractions). The release of prostaglandins into the blood can trigger a headache. Medications that counteract the actions of prostaglandin may help decrease the frequency, severity, and duration of headaches.

SCOTOMA—Scotoma is a form of aura in which the patient experiences a blind spot, of varying size, within the field of vision.

SEROTONIN—Serotonin is a chemical substance similar to histamine that is most often found in the platelets. It is believed to be prominently involved in migraine attacks. Current headache research is directed to those agents that will block the receptors for serotonin. Sumatriptan is one of this class of drugs.

TEMPORAL ARTERITIS—Temporal Arteritis (TA) refers to an inflammation of blood vessels in the temporal area of the brain. TA usually appears in patients over the age of fifty, with recent onset severe headache, often localized over the eyes. It is essential that the diagnosis be established early as temporal arteritis, because if left untreated, it can cause irreversible blindness.

TENS—Transcutaneous electrical stimulation (TENS) is a form of nondrug therapy that has been used in various pain disorders, including headaches. Similar to acupuncture, the TENS instrument attempts to stimulate nerves to block transmission of the pain impulses to the spinal cord. The results in headache therapy have been negligible.

TENSION-TYPE HEADACHE—These headaches are thus called because emotional factors such as stress are believed to be their triggers. These headaches may be accompanied by pain in the neck and shoulders. They are caused by tightening of the muscles at the back of the neck and of the face and scalp. There are two types of tension-type headaches, episodic and chronic. The episodic form is easily controlled with over-the-counter analgesics. In the chronic form the headaches occur on a daily or almost daily basis. In both forms the headaches are two-sided and are often described as a tight band or a vise-like ache. Chronic tension-type headaches can be due to anxiety or depression.

Treatment of the acute headache should be limited to mild, non-habituating analgesics. For prevention of the chronic form, the cause of the headaches must be determined. Chronic tension-type headaches due to anxiety are best treated with a mild tranquilizing agent, buspirone. For those headaches due to depression, the antidepressants are the drugs of choice in preventive treatment.

TOXIC VASCULAR HEADACHE—Some patients will experience headaches due to external factors. The toxic headache includes headaches due to poor ventilation, reactions with foods or drugs, or fever. Headache is a common symptom for those exposed to high levels of carbon monoxide or nitrates (such as workers in munitions plants). Foods containing nitrites, such as hot dogs, may trigger a headache. Fever may cause a severe headache, and a potentially serious case should not be ruled out in these patients.

TRANQUILIZERS—Tranquilizers usually are not used in headache treatment by most specialists. These medications are used in the treatment of anxiety and other emotional disorders. Many of these drugs are habit-forming and in elderly patients can cause serious side effects.

TYRAMINE—Tyramine is a naturally occurring substance in certain foods. It is called vasoactive as it can cause the blood vessels to expand and thus trigger a headache, such as migraine. Tyramine is found in a variety of foods, including aged cheese, nuts, yogurt, and is also found in alcoholic beverages. All headache patients should receive a tyramine-restricted diet to determine if avoiding these foods will decrease their headaches.

VASOCONSTRICTION—Vasoconstriction refers to a decrease in the size of the blood vessels.

VASODILATION—Vasodilation refers to an increase in the size of the blood vessels.

WARNINGS OF MIGRAINE—These are vague symptoms that precede migraine without aura. They include fatigue or surge of energy, an increase or loss of appetite, restlessness, or listlessness.

*I*NDEX

Abdominal migraine, 125, 193,
  201
Acetaminophen, 58–59, 129, 134,
  145
ACTH (adrenal-cortex-stimulating
  hormone), 35, 115
Acupuncture, 152, 172, 193
Adrenal gland, 32, 34, 35, 39–41,
  100, 113–14, 115, 116, 124,
  157, 176
Adrenaline (epinephrine), 39, 114,
  116, 124, 157, 176, 195
Age, of onset of headaches, 7–9,
  24, 42, 47, 66, 122–23. *See
  also* Children's headaches
Alcoholic beverages, 5, 39, 108,
  175–76, 207
Allergies, 19, 43
Alpha agonists, 142, 193
Amines. *See* Vasoactive amines
Analgesics. *See* Pain relievers
Androgens, 40, 41
Aneurysms, 3, 18, 23, 117, 193–94
Angiography, 86–87
Anovulation therapy, 59

Antidepressants, 105–6, 107, 110,
  135–36, 143, 194, 198, 207
  MAOIs, 108, 110, 136, 202
Anxiety, 14, 15, 88, 155. *See also*
  Depression; Stress
  sexual headaches and, 113–14
Anxiety headaches, 10, 16, 101,
  102, 104, 106, 109–10, 194
  in children, 124
  diagnosing of, 6–21
  treatment of, 108
Arteritis, temporal (TA), 23, 206
Aspartame, 178
Aspirin, 5, 20, 58, 101, 129, 134,
  139, 140, 141, 143, 144,
  145, 147, 203
  prostaglandins and, 57, 99–100,
  139, 143
Aura, 13–14, 48, 56, 63–65, 68,
  70, 72, 74, 75, 78, 125, 126,
  139, 150, 151, 194, 201
  in children's headaches, 123
  hormone-replacement therapy
  and, 90–91
  scotoma, 206